So What? Now What?

Osher Günsberg

So What? Now What?

How to stop being stuck and start living!

illustrated by Campbell Walker aka Struthless

I can't stand this any longer.

Nothing **ever** goes right.

It's one bad thing after the next.

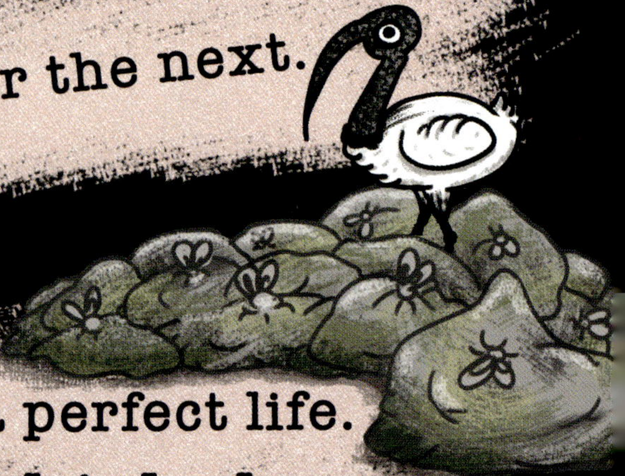

Everyone else has a perfect life.

My life is a rubbish dump.

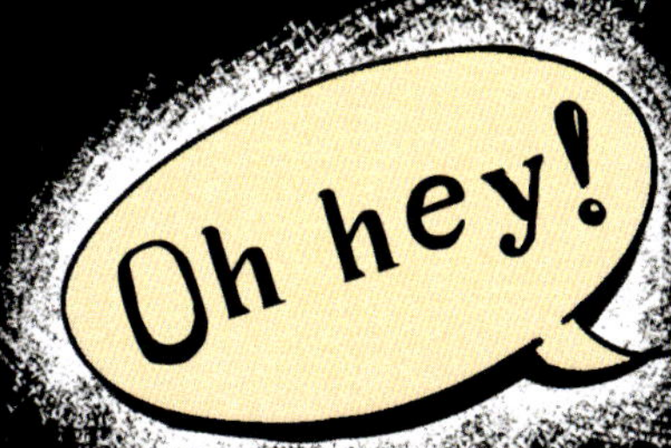

What you're going through sounds really rough.

And what are **you** supposed to be?

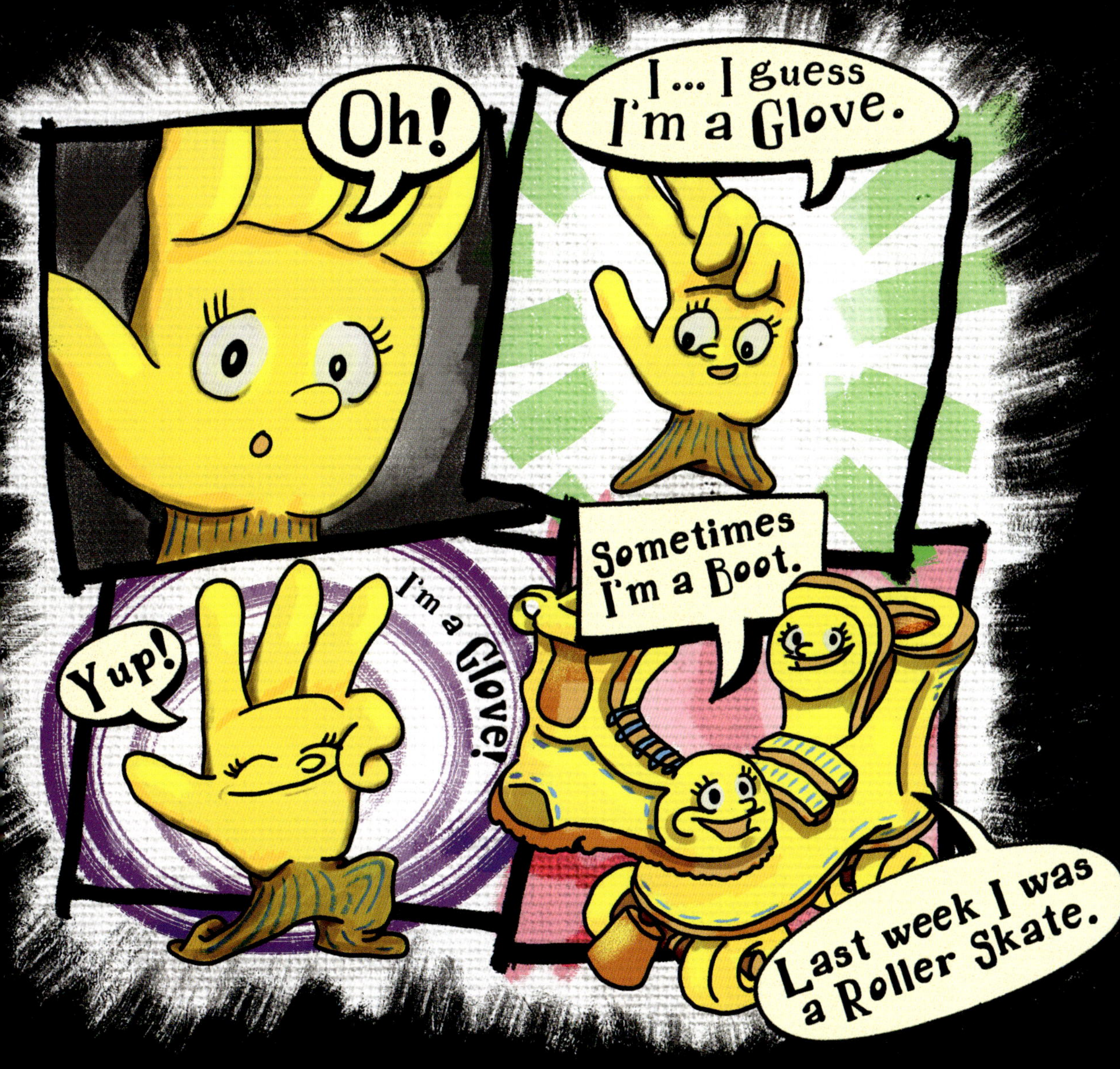
Oh!
I... I guess I'm a Glove.
Yup!
I'm a Glove!
Sometimes I'm a Boot.
Last week I was a Roller Skate.

What do *you* want?

I get what's happening to you, and I might be able to show you a path out of the discomfort.

Spare me.

How could a ***cartoon glove*** in a book make ***anything*** better?

SMÅÅSHE
You're right;
it won't.
A set of instructions won't
build your flatpack couch

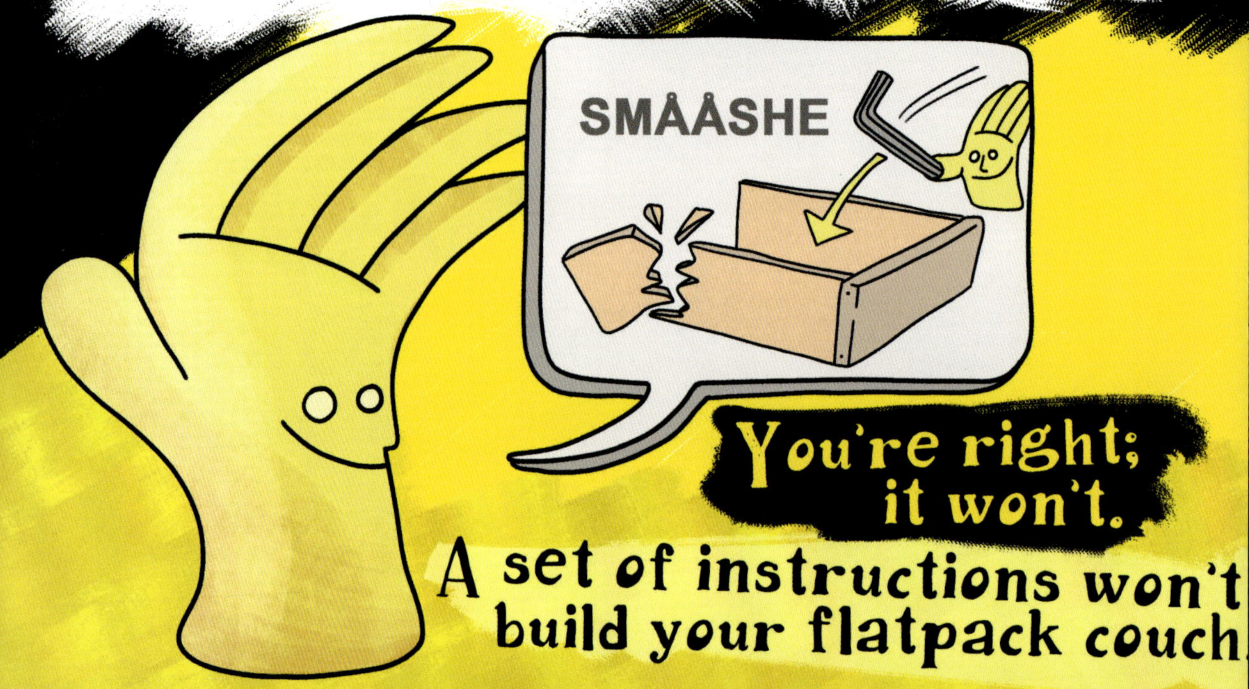

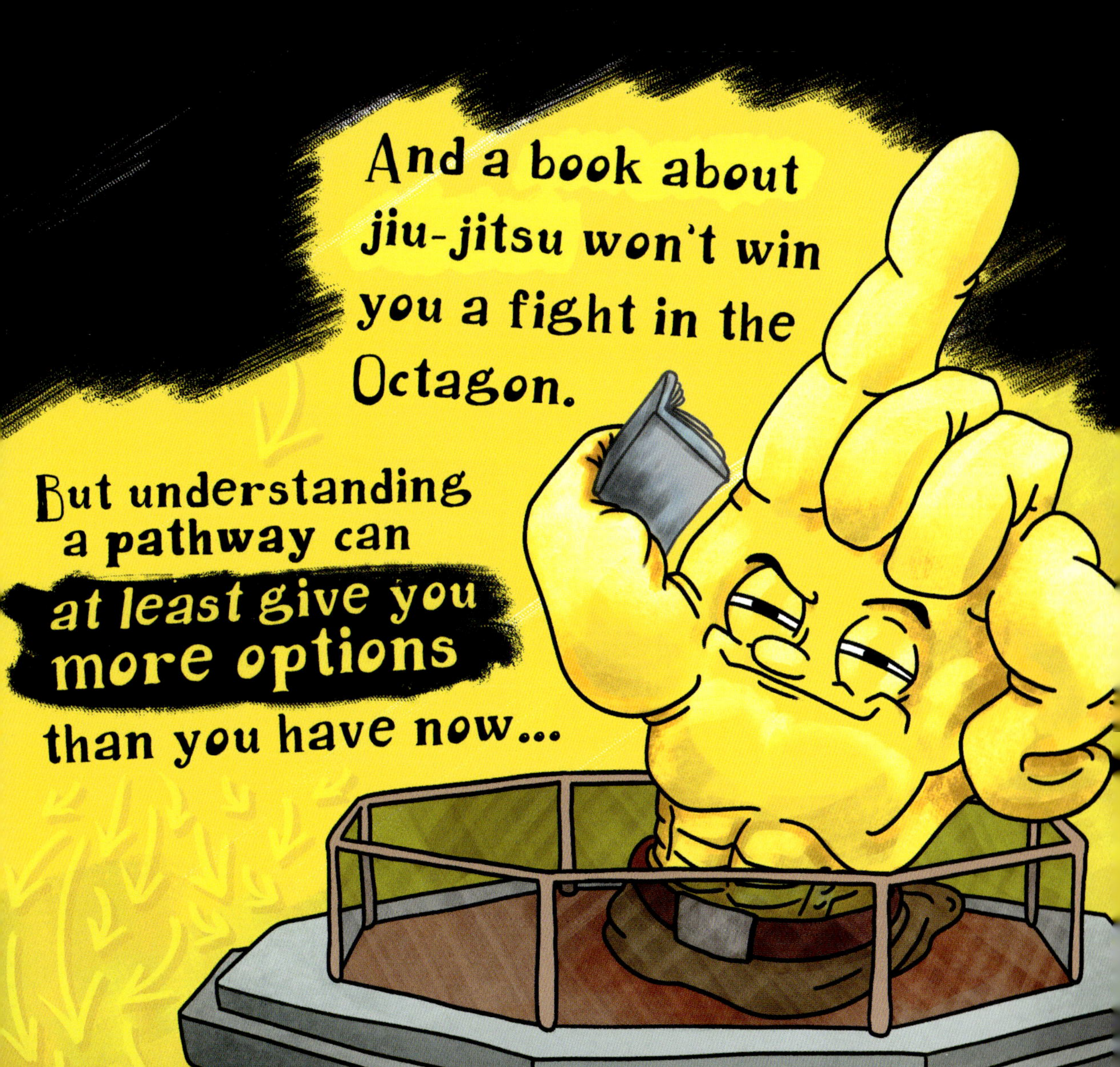
And a book about jiu-jitsu won't win you a fight in the Octagon.
But understanding a pathway can at least give you more options than you have now...

You heard how **bad** things are on page one.

It's like I have **no control** over my life.

What kind of goal could I ***possibly achieve*** when I feel so powerless?

We each have a place we want to move towards, and how it looks is different for all of us.

Goals can be things like

health, relationships, and financial security. family, work

But they could also be none of those things.

You're just making me feel worse.

I've tried ***everything*** to have things like that in my life,

but **every time I try,** I get smashed down again and again and again.

Each time it hurts more, and nothing I try is making the pain go away.

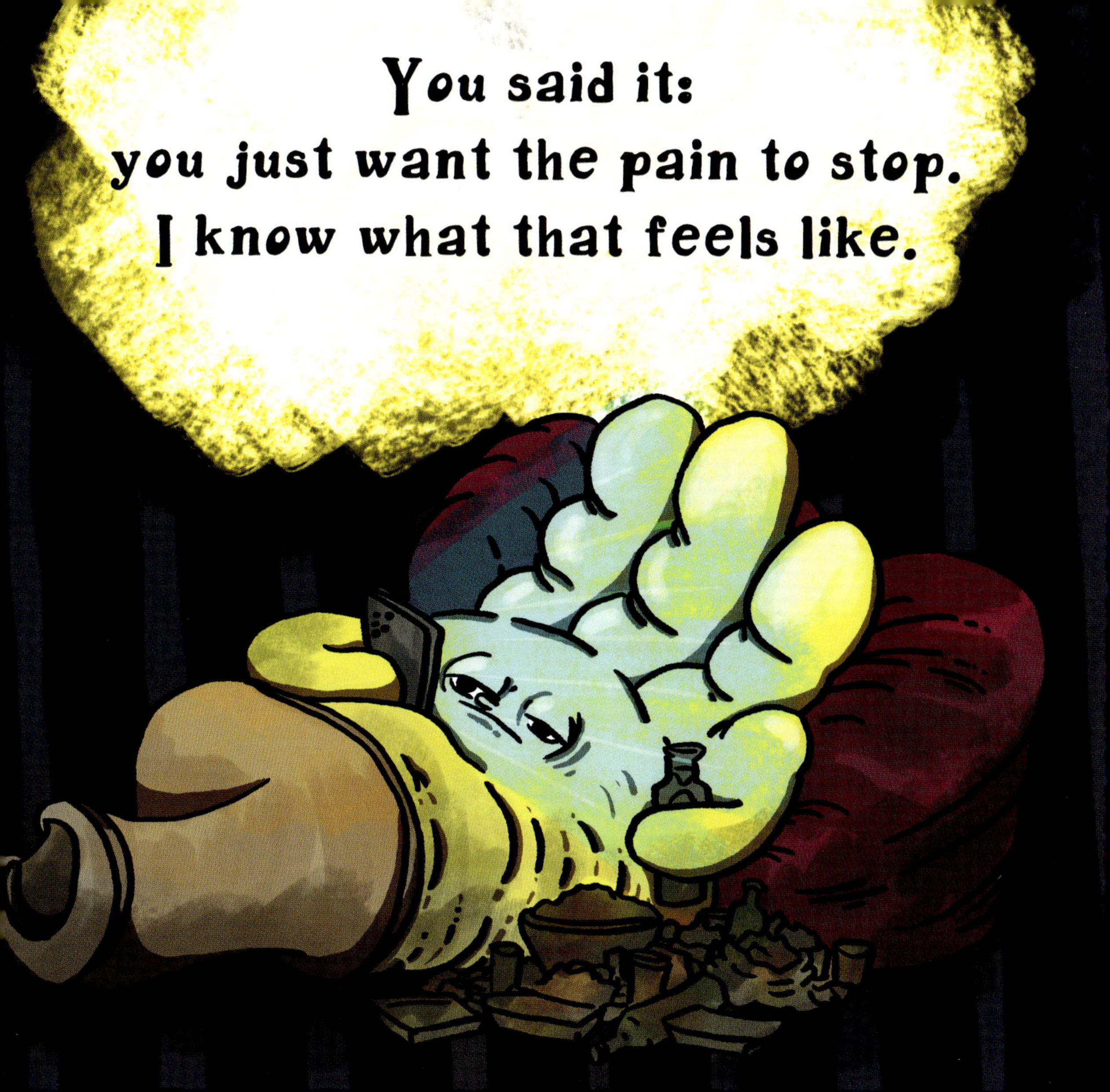
You said it:
you just want the pain to stop.
I know what that feels like.

You have **no idea** how I feel now.
Nobody understands.

Not even your friends?

They're **too busy** living their **perfect lives.**

They used to ask me how I'm doing
but one by one they stopped.
The last one to abandon me was my ex.

If they asked now, would you have a different answer?

No.

The only thing that's changed is how often things go badly. It's constant.

Sounds like you're pretty stuck.

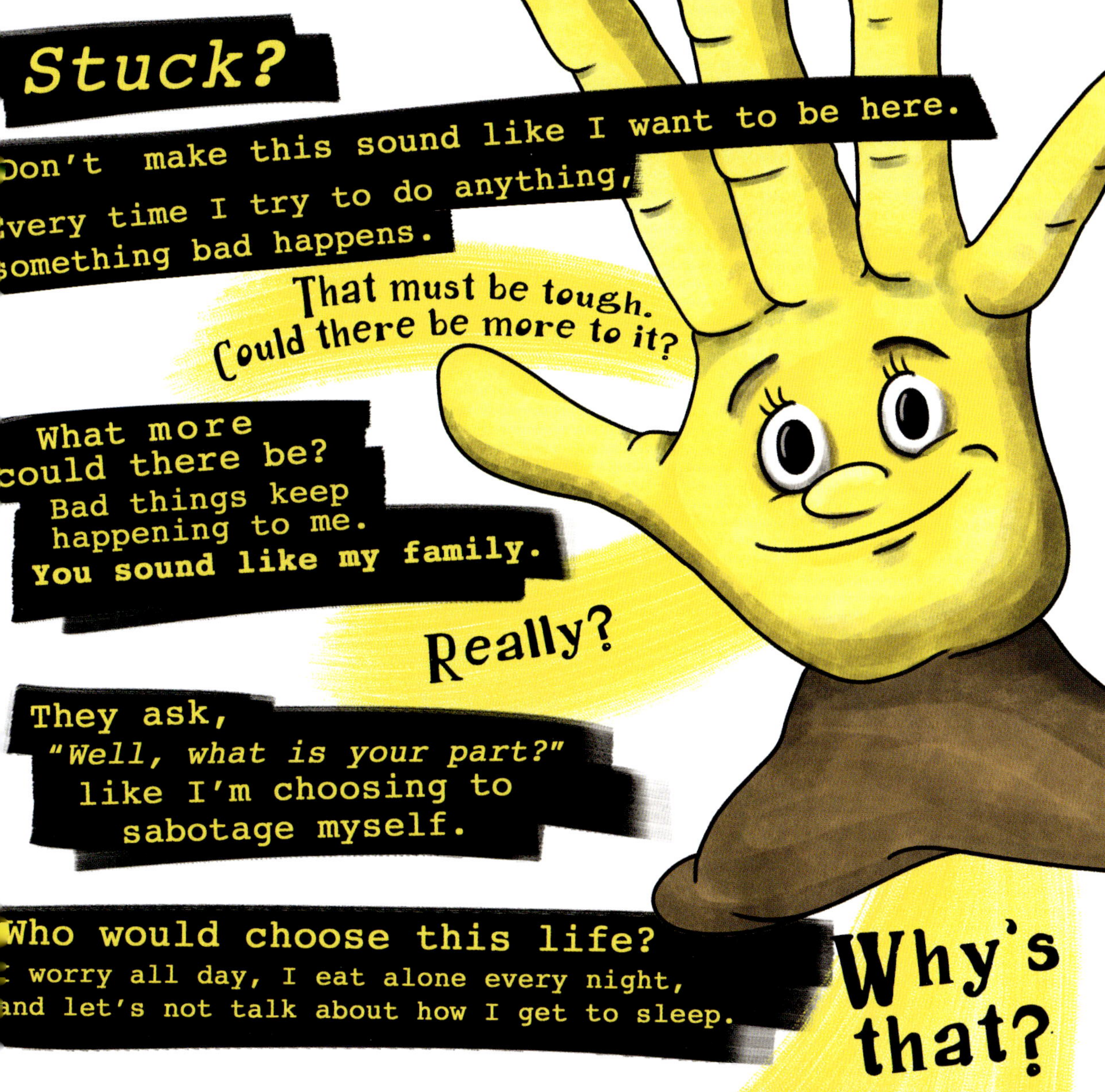
Stuck?
Don't make this sound like I want to be here.
Every time I try to do anything,
something bad happens.
That must be tough.
Could there be more to it?
What more
could there be?
Bad things keep
happening to me.
You sound like my family.
Really?
They ask,
"Well, what is your part?"
like I'm choosing to
sabotage myself.
Who would choose this life?
I worry all day, I eat alone every night,
and let's not talk about how I get to sleep.
Why's
that?

Let's just say
the things that used to numb the pain
don't even touch the sides now.
It used to be just at night,
but now it's **earlier and earlier every day.**

Sometimes even at work.

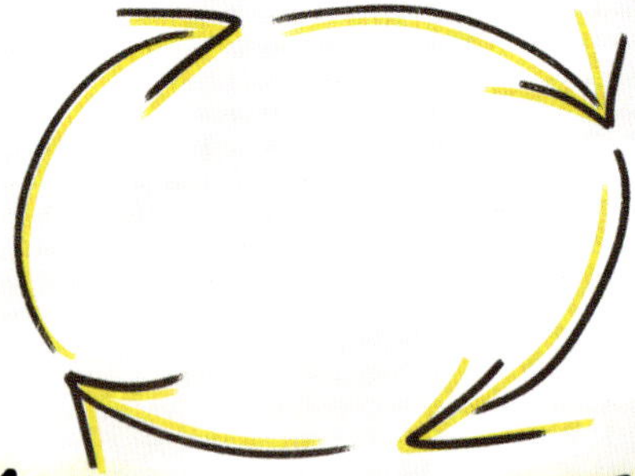

At first it helps,
but eventually the amount you need
to feel something **close to okay**
causes **more** and **more damage.**

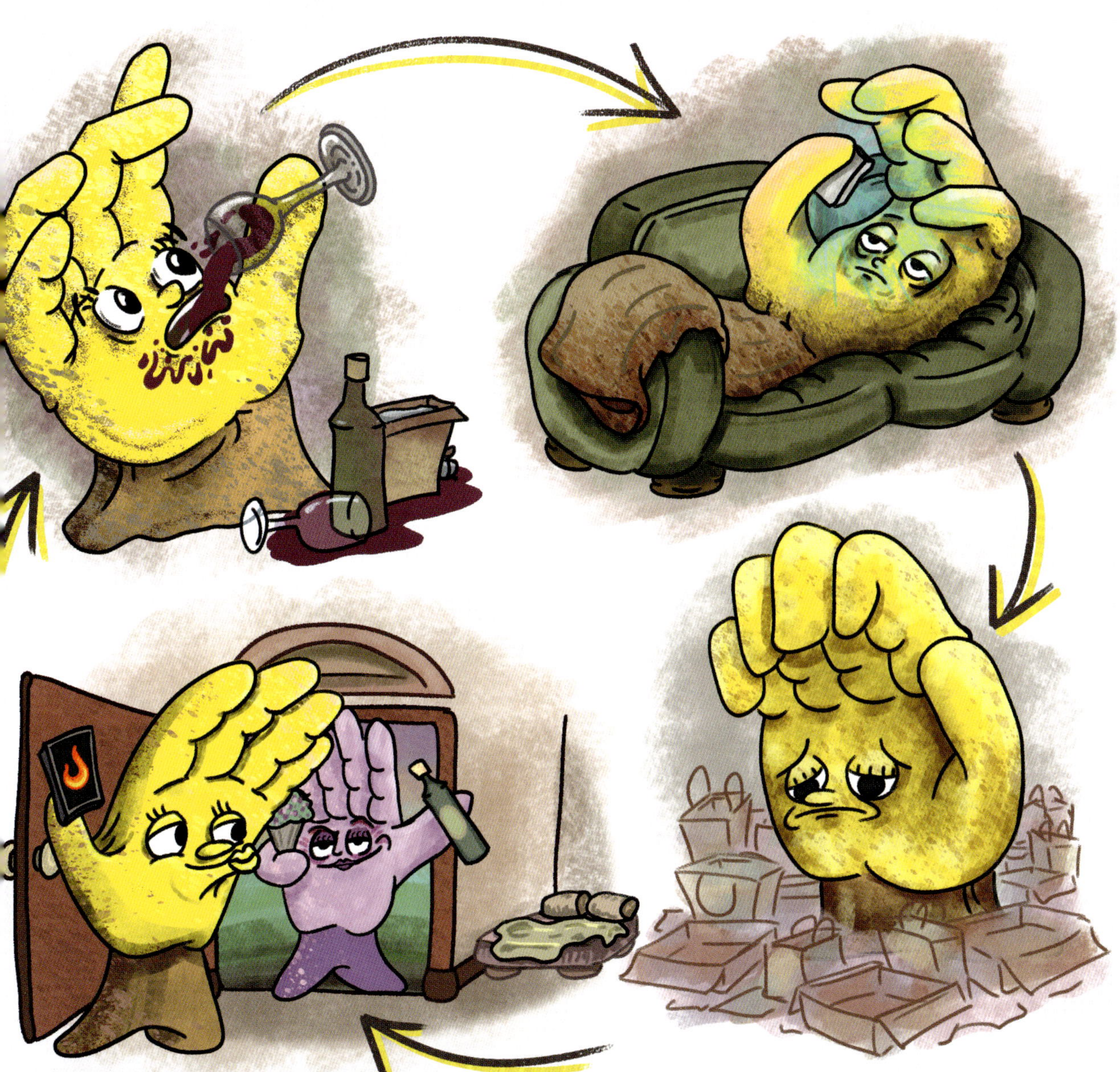

And how would you know?

Because I've been where you are.
I was lucky to come out the other side.

Oh good for you!!

You weren't dealing with **what I'm dealing with.**

It doesn't matter what I was dealing with.
What matters is that I was exactly where you are now.
Stuck in blame and stuck in pain.

Seriously?

You sound like a **cheesy couch cushion.**
Do you *always* speak in rhymes?

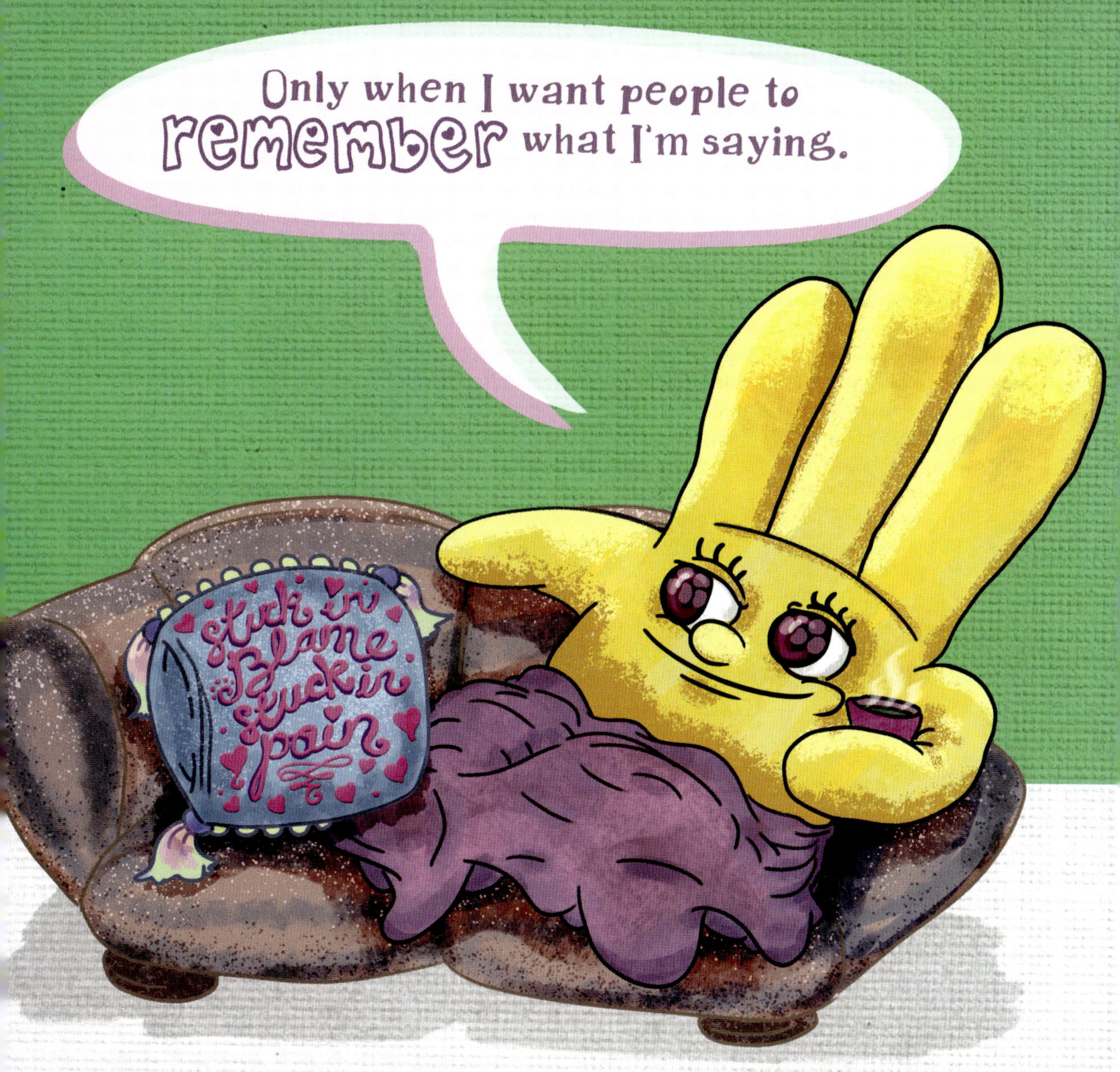
Only when I want people to
remember what I'm saying.
stuck in
Blame
stuck in
pain

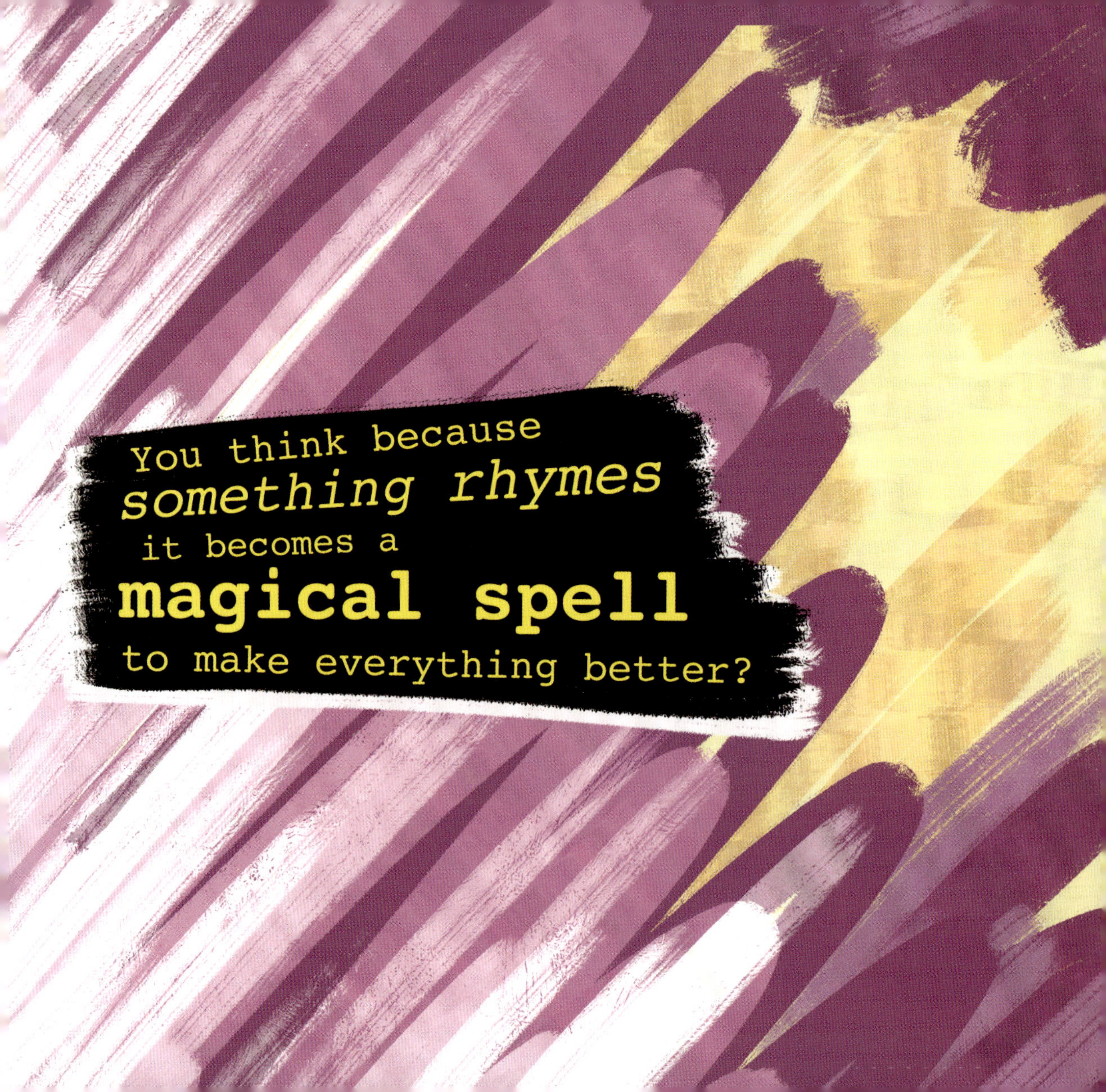
You think because
something rhymes
it becomes a
magical spell
to make everything better?

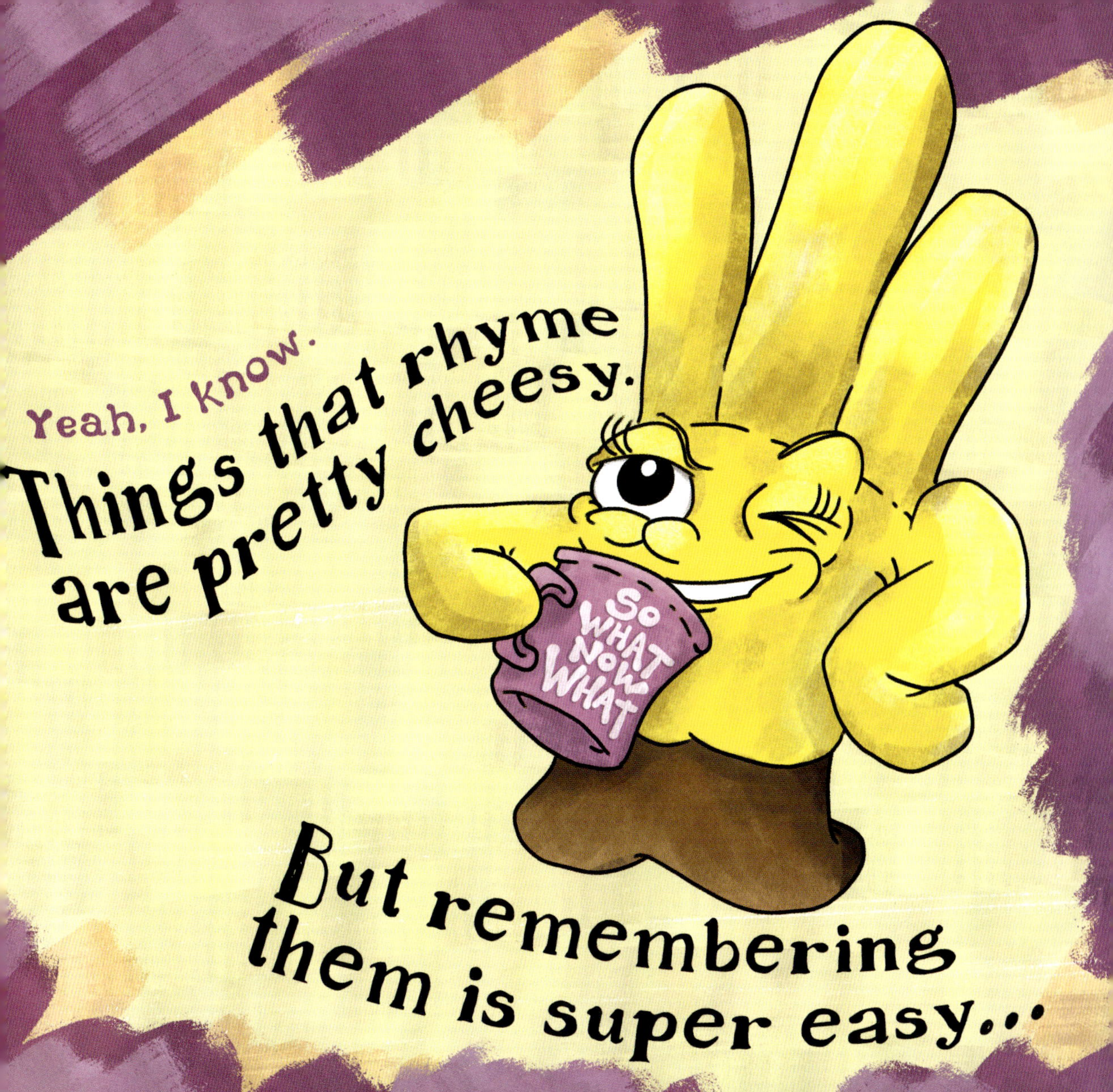
Yeah, I know.
Things that rhyme are pretty cheesy.
SO WHAT NOW WHAT
But remembering them is super easy...

If searching for blame is bad, how else do I describe who's at fault for all of this?

Why does it matter?

Because **someone** has to pay for my life going down the toilet.

And what would change if there was a way to make "someone" pay?

I'd feast on the delicious taste of

vindicating revenge!

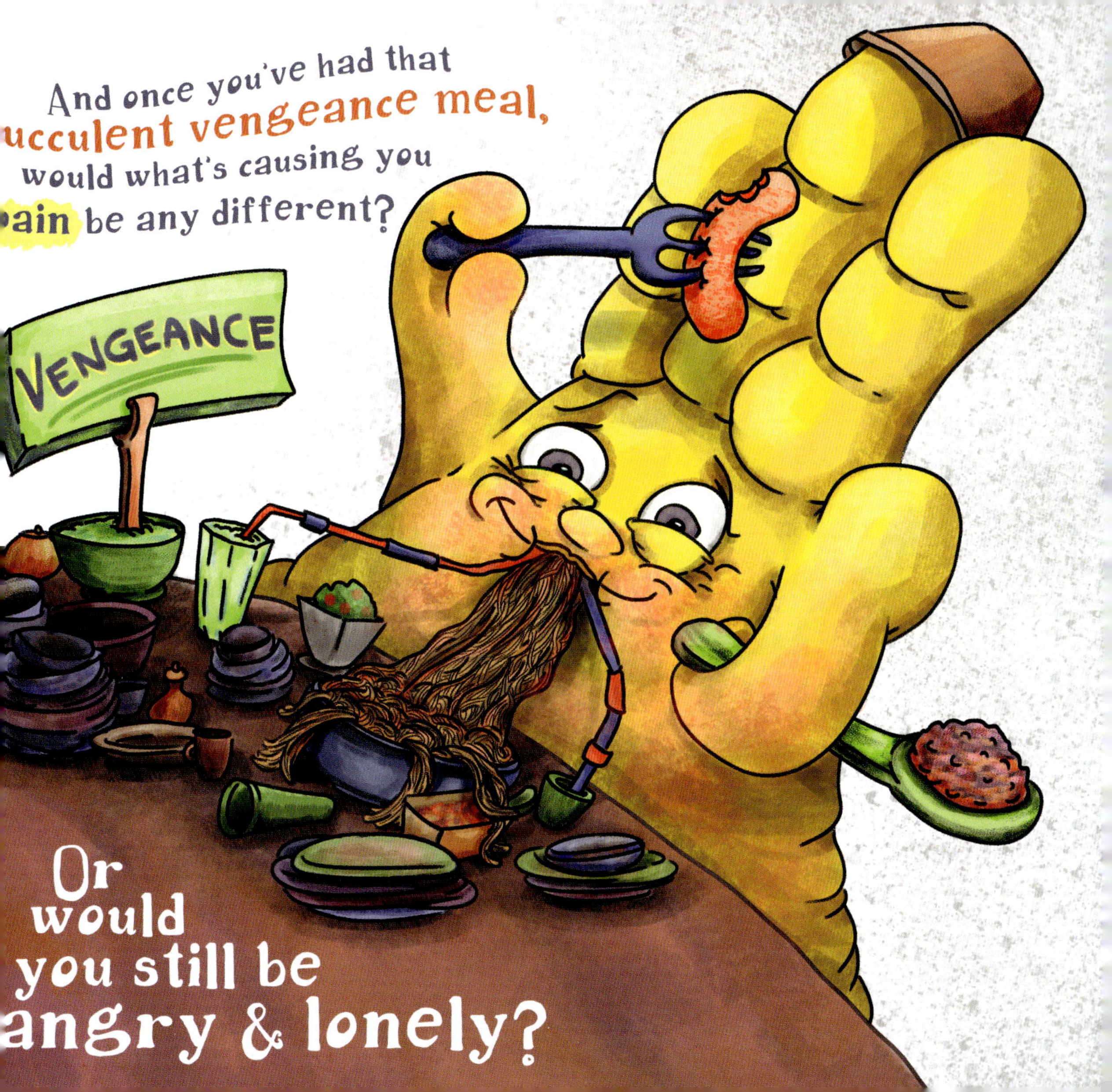
And once you've had that
ucculent vengeance meal,
would what's causing you
ain be any different?
VENGEANCE
Or
would
you still be
angry & lonely?

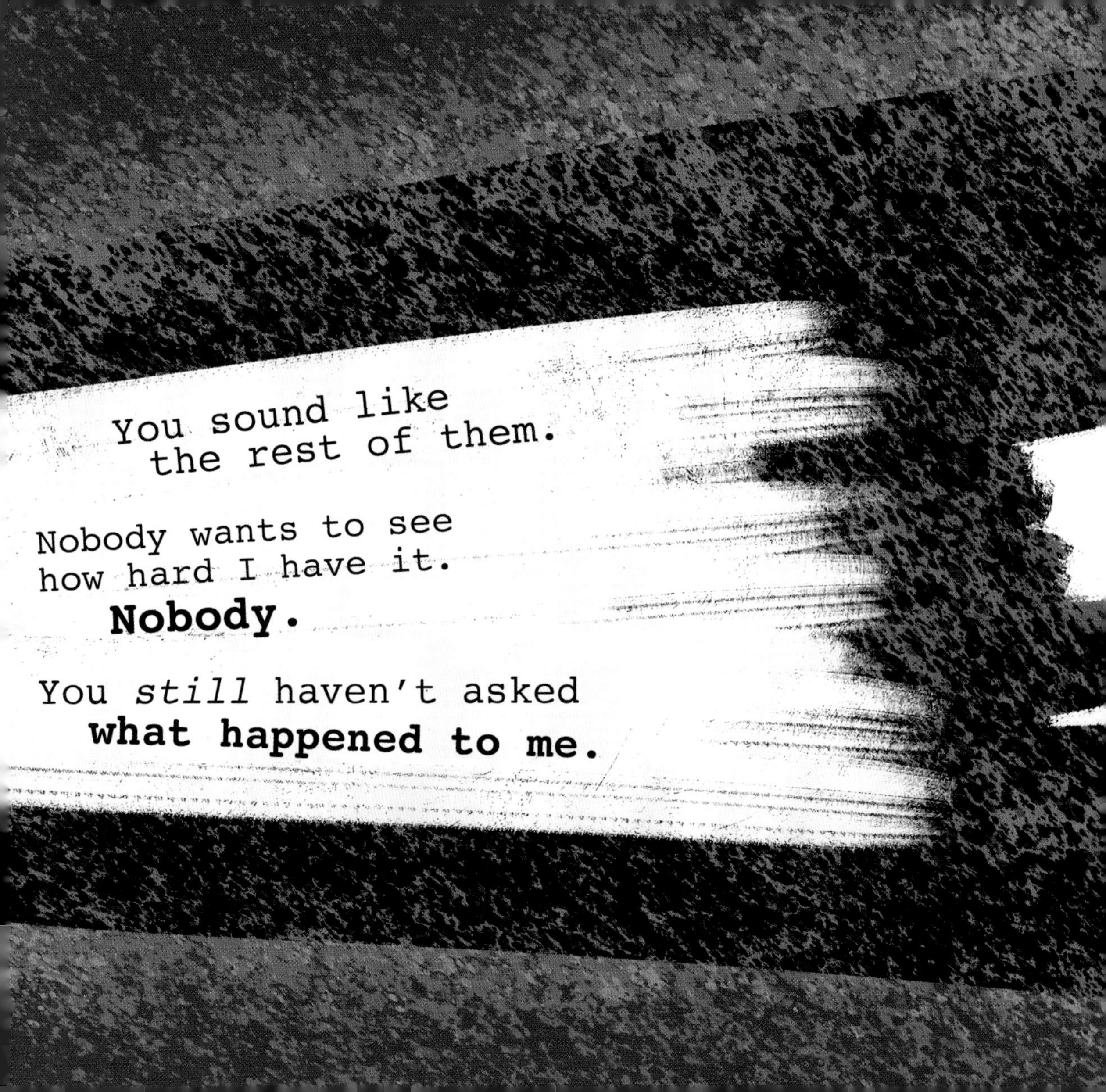
You sound like
the rest of them.
Nobody wants to see
how hard I have it.
Nobody.
You *still* haven't asked
what happened to me.

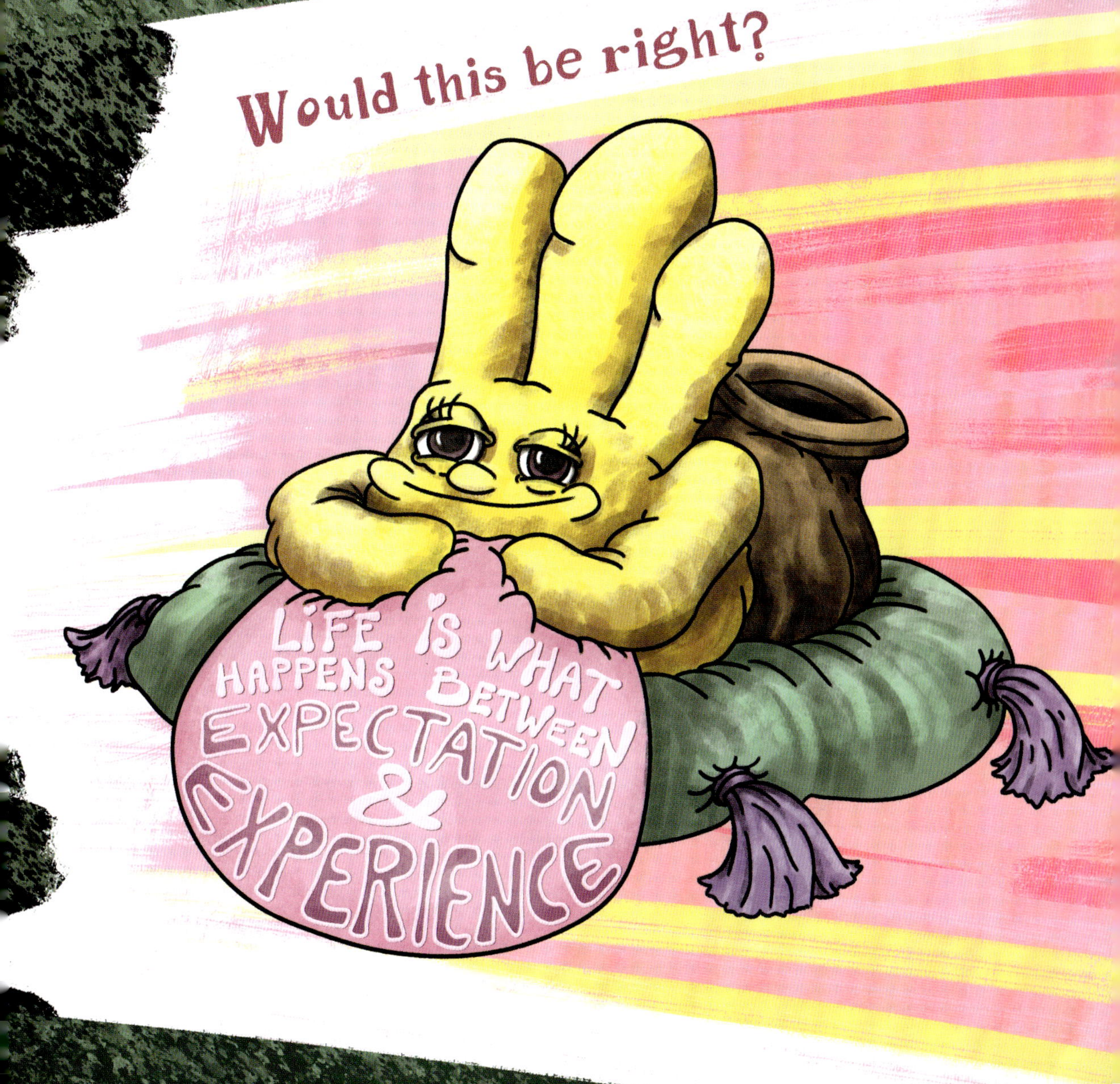
Would this be right?
LIFE IS WHAT HAPPENS BETWEEN EXPECTATION & EXPERIENCE

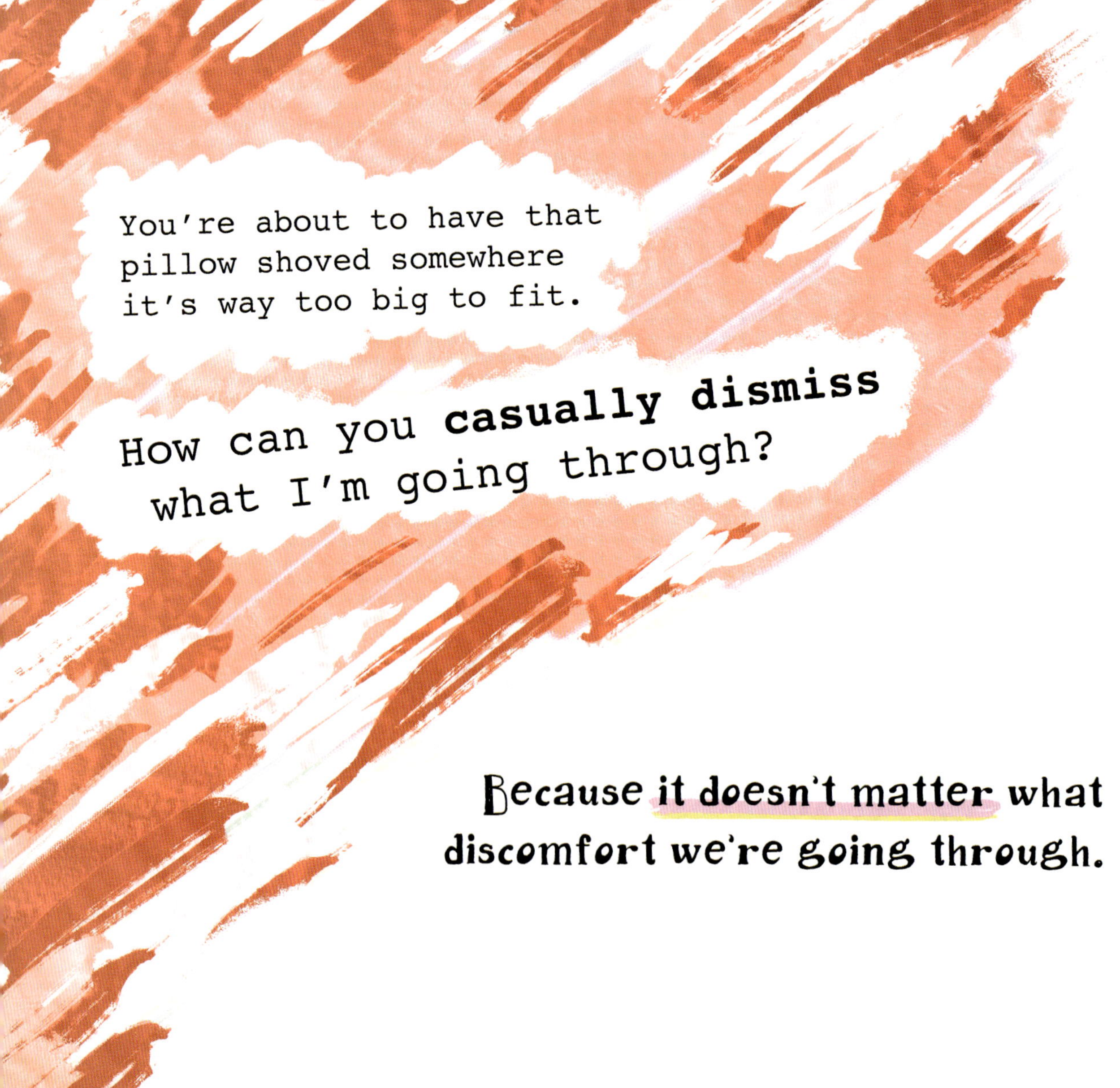

Because it doesn't matter what discomfort we're going through.

The gap between expectation and experience always matches what we feel.

You expected to be in love forever.
They felt differently.
You broke up.

You expected to be healthy.
Now the doctor wants to order more tests because they're worried about something.

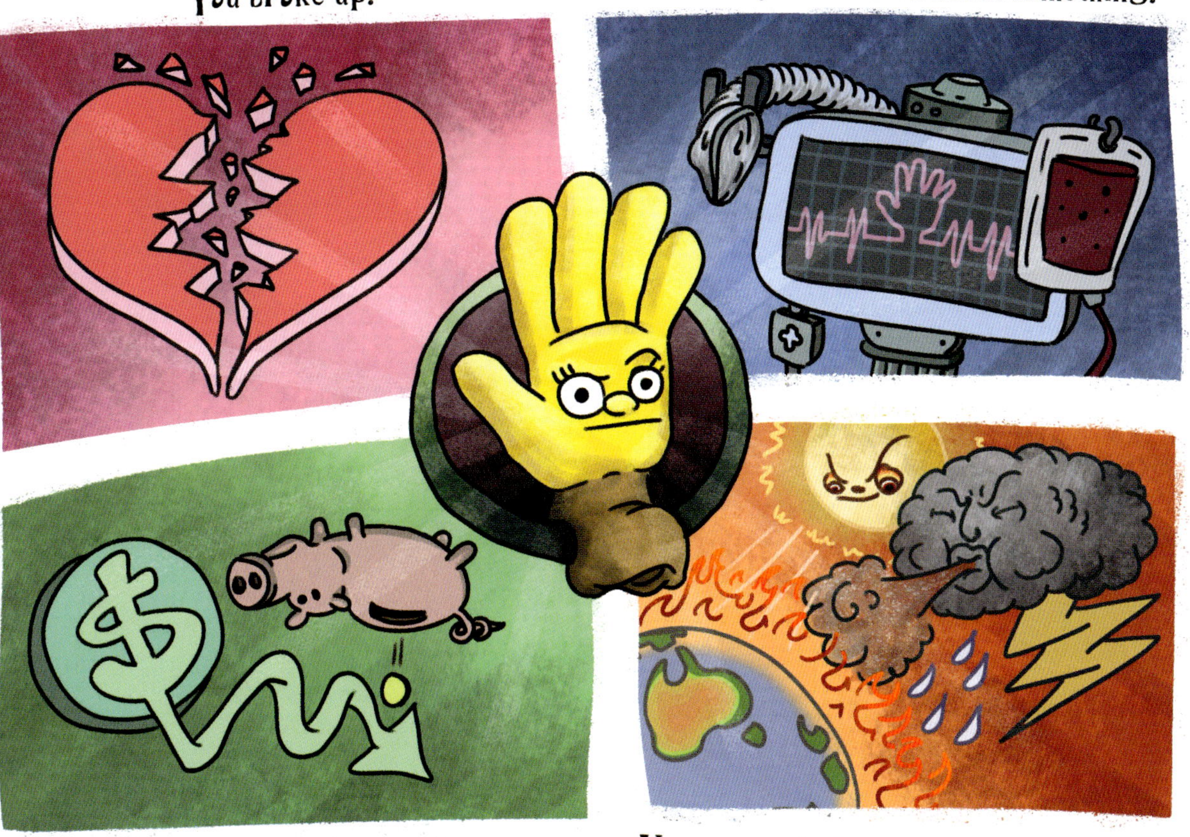

You expected job security.
The economy tanked and now you're unemployed.

You expected a predictable future.
We've cooked the climate so much it isn't looking good.

Does any of this sound familiar?

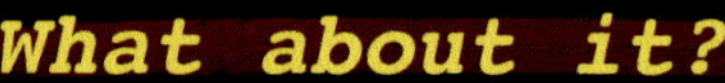

Every one of those things is beyond our control. That kind of pain is inescapable.

I disagree. Between expectation and experience, which can you control?

THIS IS **INFURIATING.** I'm about to **stop reading** if this keeps up.

That's okay. It's an uncomfortable idea. Our sense of self can try to protect us in all kinds of ways...

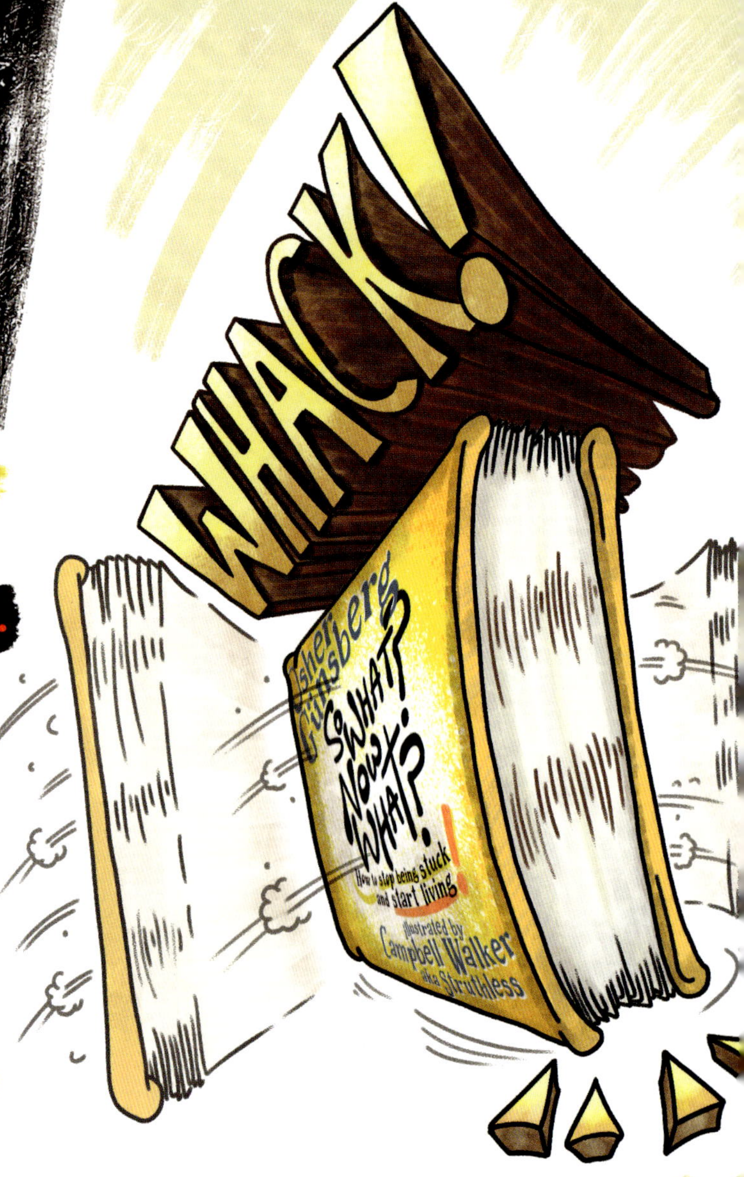

WHACK!

Usher Ginsberg
So What? Now What?!
How to stop being stuck and start living
Illustrated by Campbell Walker aka Struthless

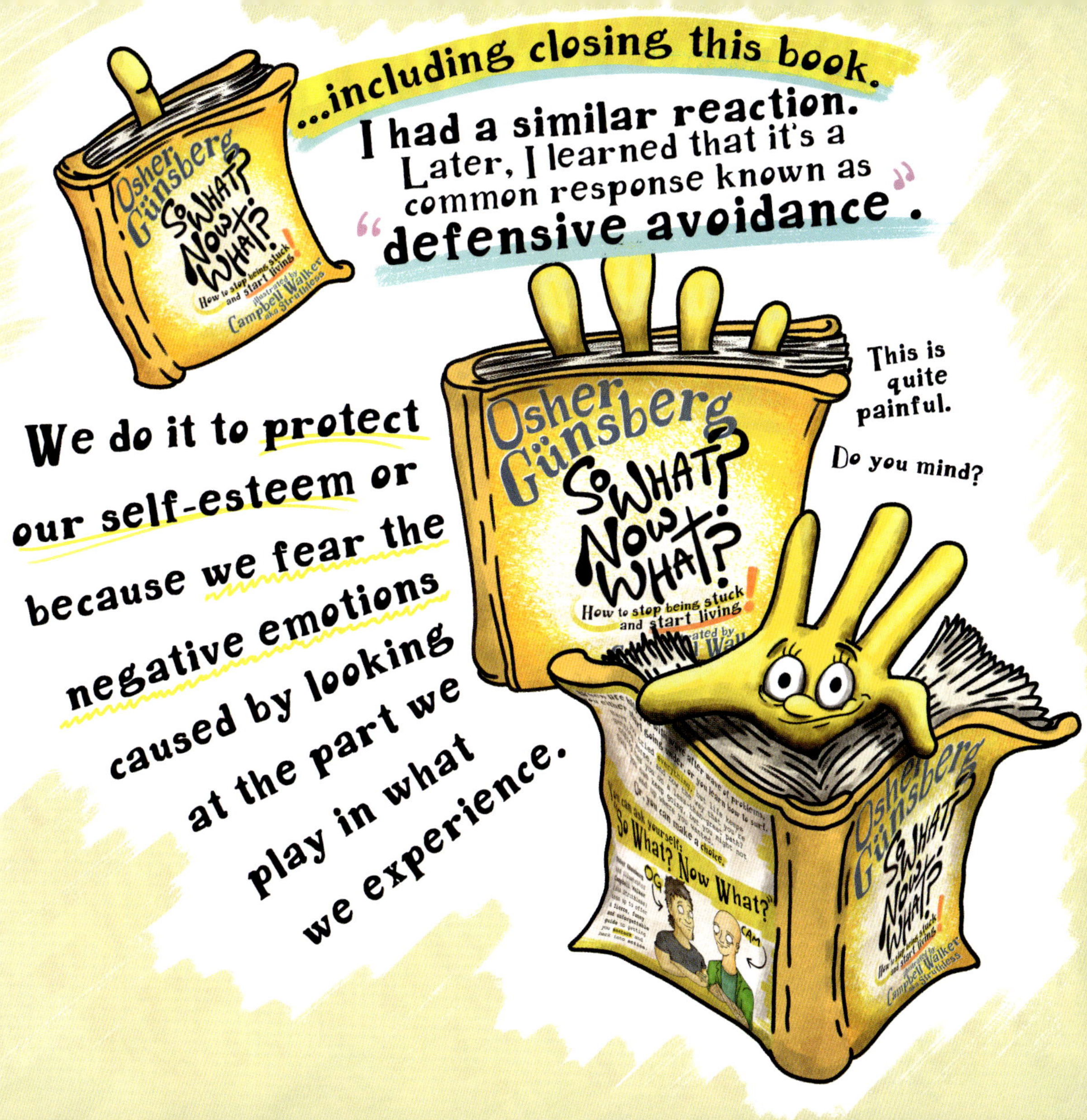
...including closing this book.
I had a similar reaction.
Later, I learned that it's a
common response known as
"defensive avoidance".
This is
quite
painful.
Do you mind?
We do it to protect
our self-esteem or
because we fear the
negative emotions
caused by looking
at the part we
play in what
we experience.

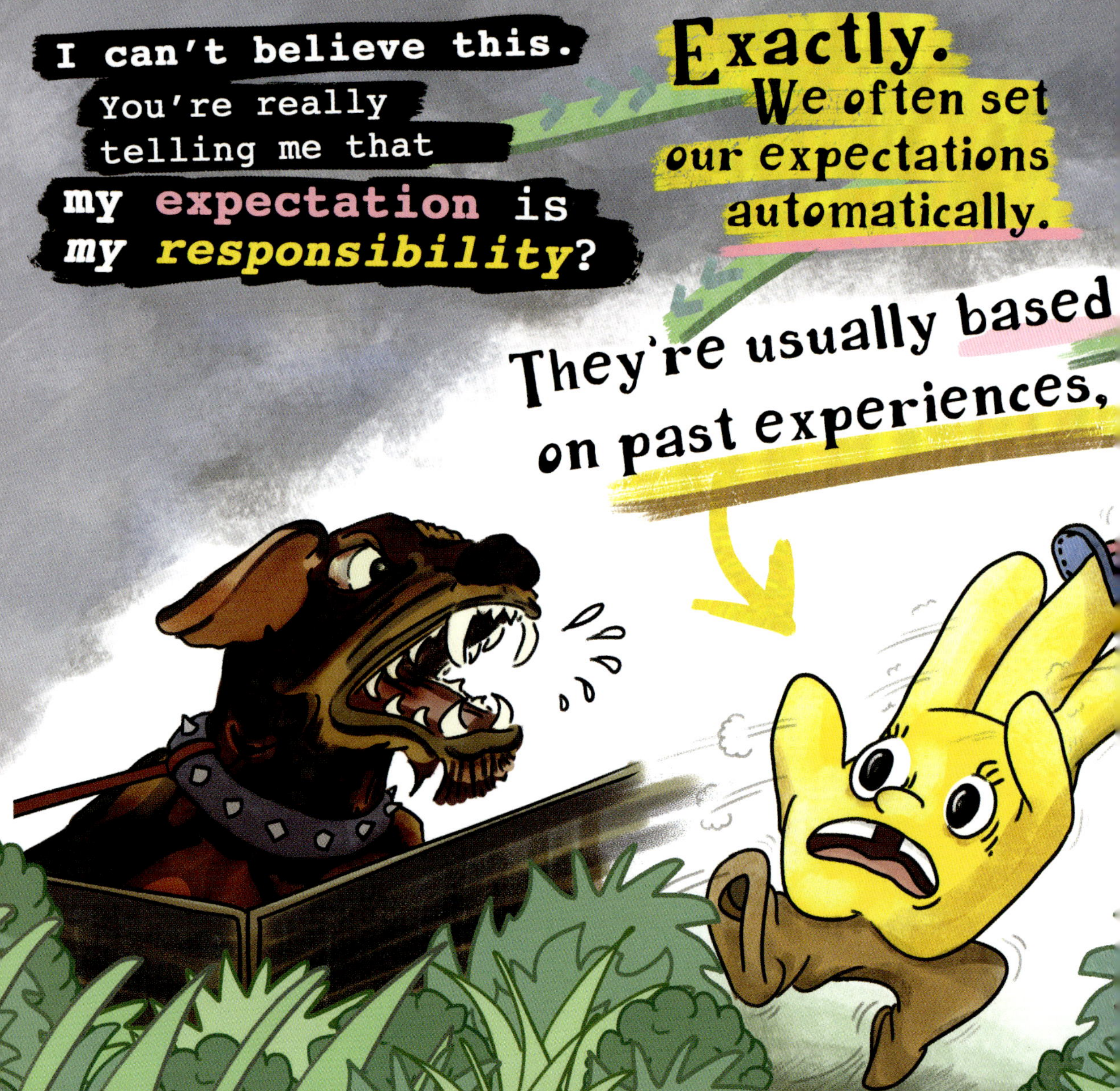
I can't believe this.
You're really telling me that my expectation is my responsibility?
Exactly.
We often set our expectations automatically.
They're usually based on past experiences,

It can happen so quickly we don't even realise we've done it.

possibly unrelated to what's happening right now.

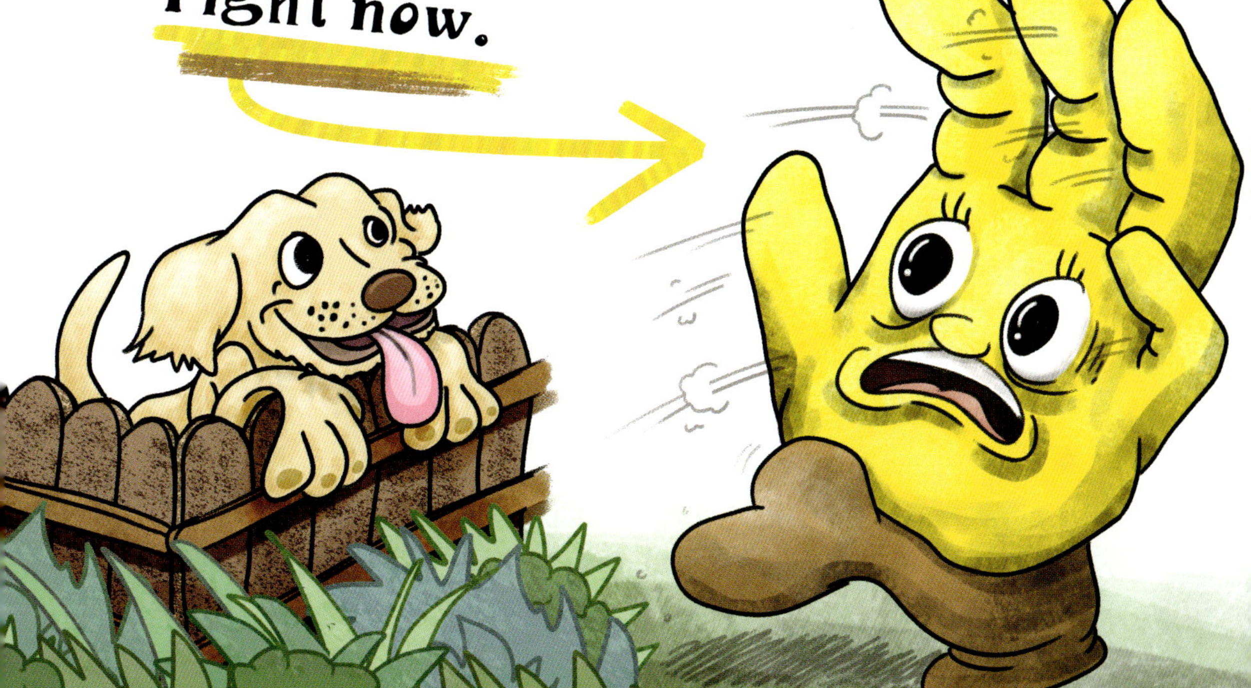

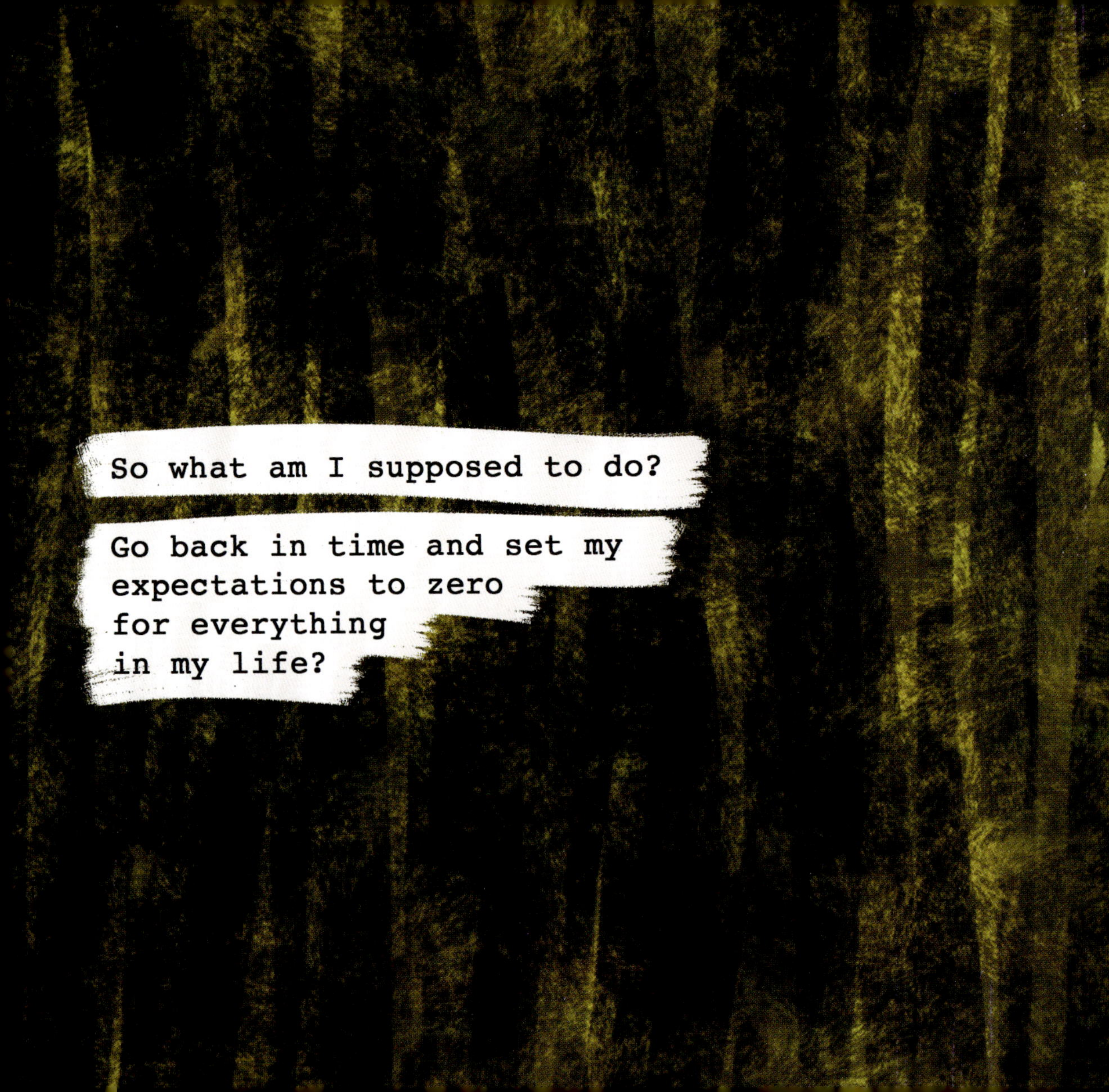
So what am I supposed to do?
Go back in time and set my
expectations to zero
for everything
in my life?

As far as I'm aware,

there's no time machine

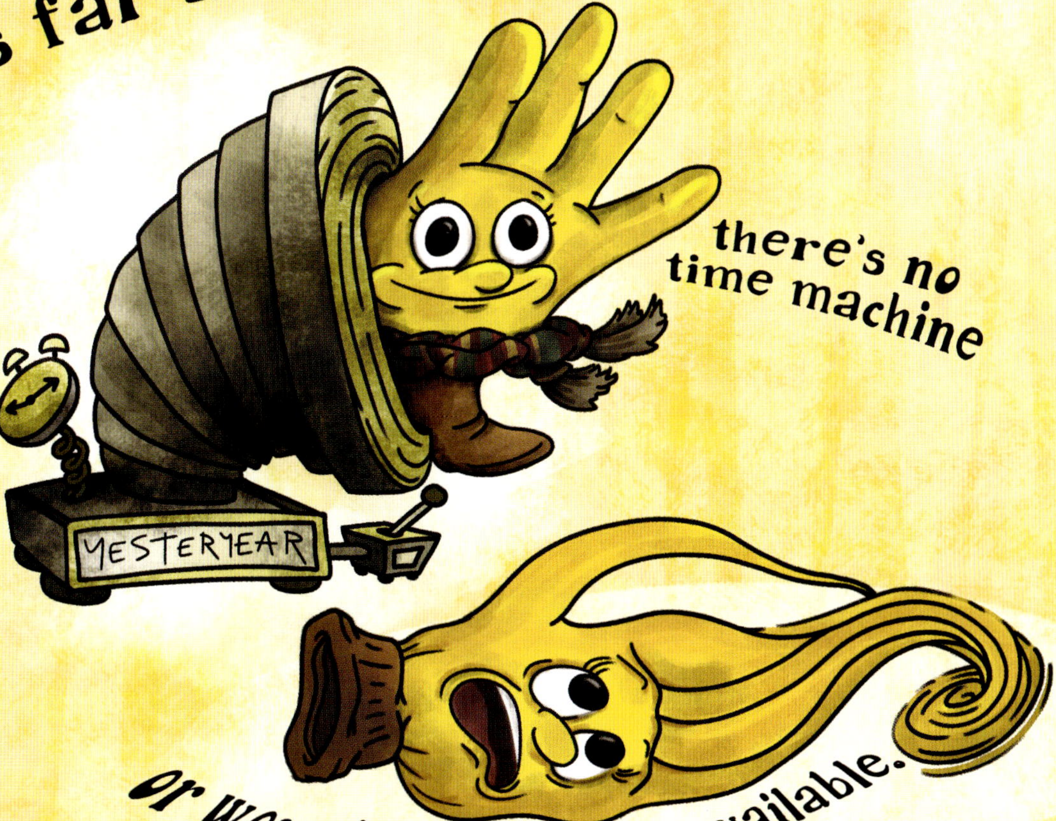

or wormhole currently available.

But I've got the next best thing.

Just get to your point, please.

SHAME
ANGUISH
PAIN
FEAR
DOOM
PANIC
You're telling me that life is unbearable. You can't control what's happening.

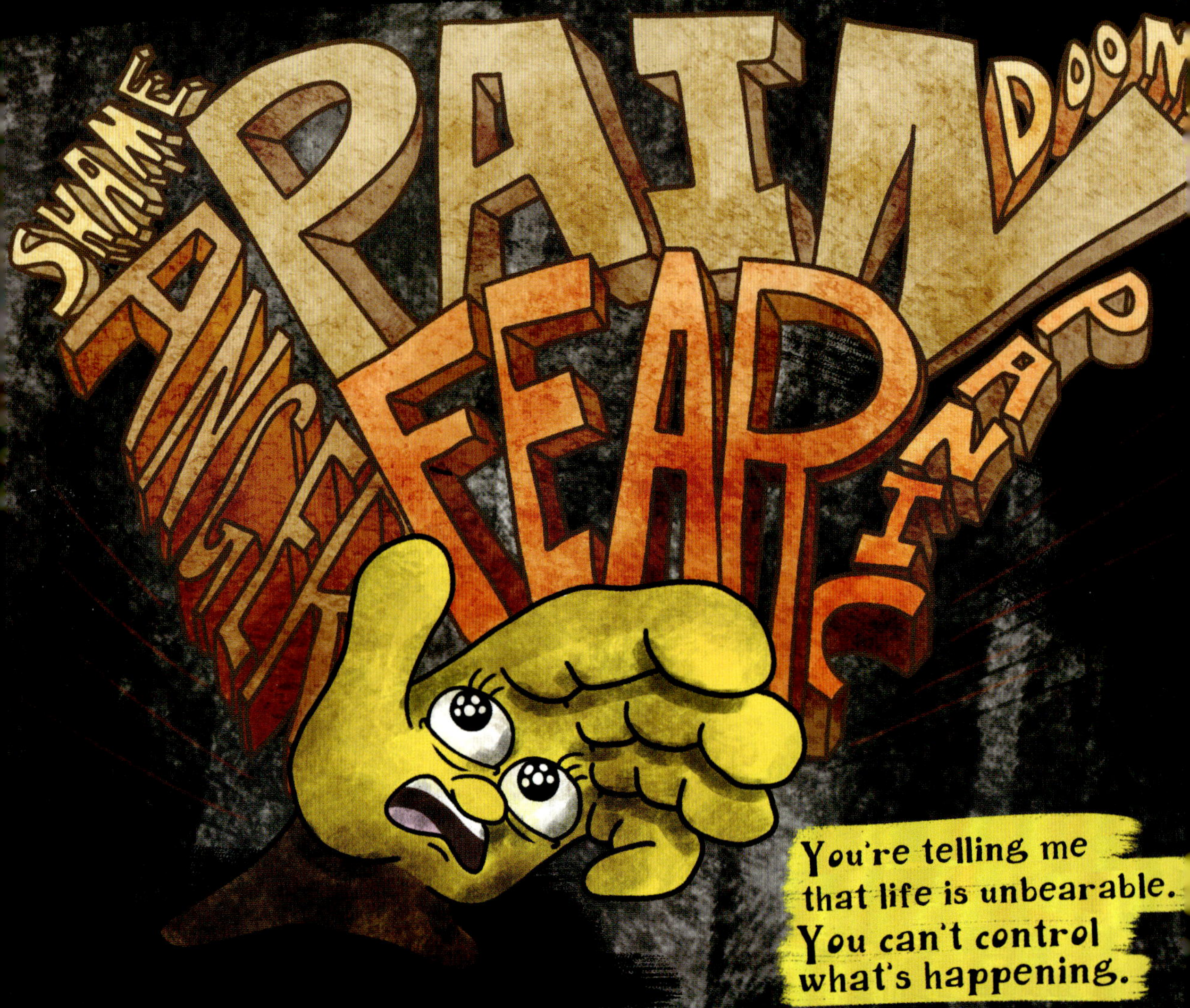

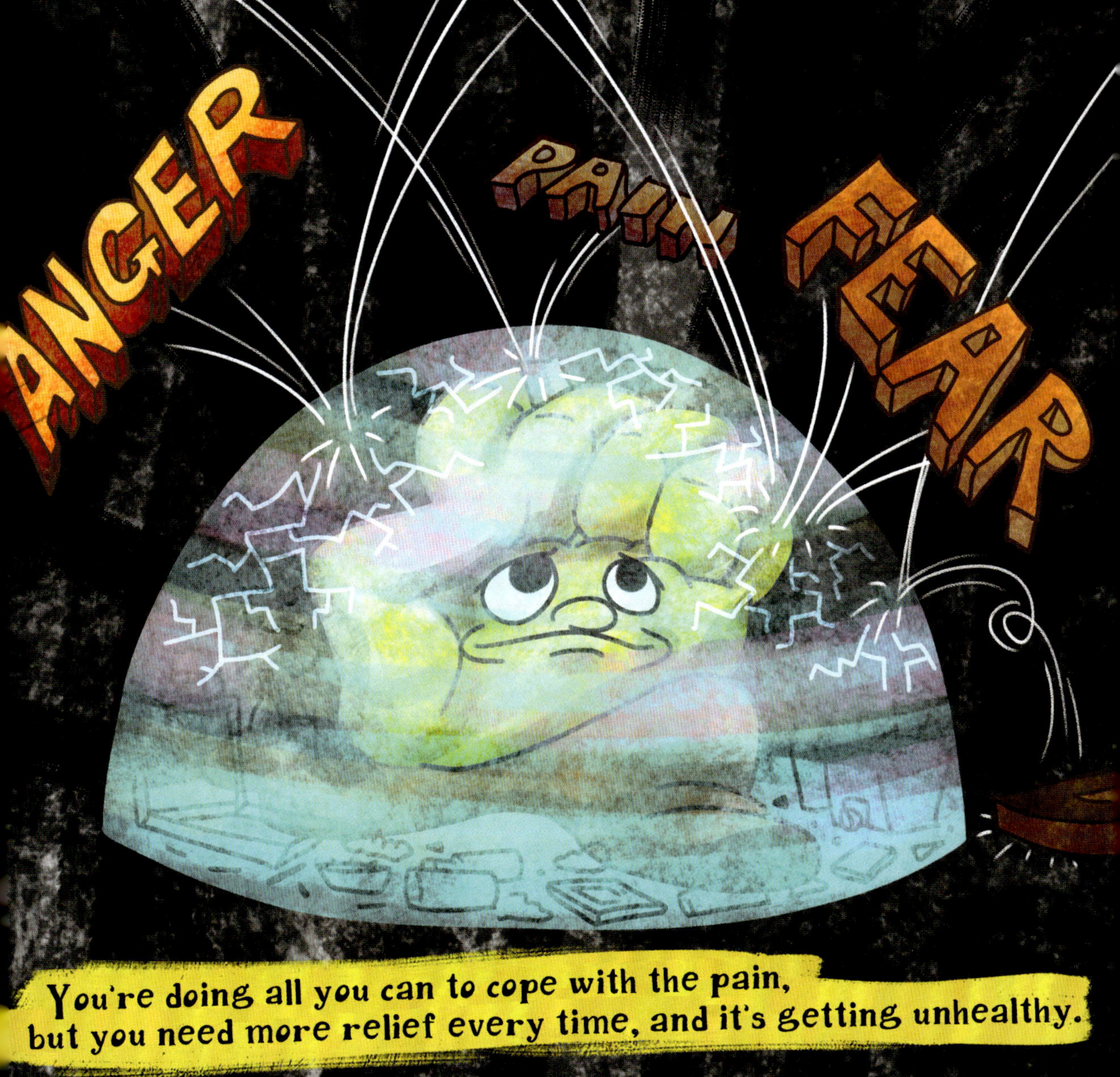
ANGER
PAIN
FEAR
You're doing all you can to cope with the pain,
but you need more relief every time, and it's getting unhealthy.

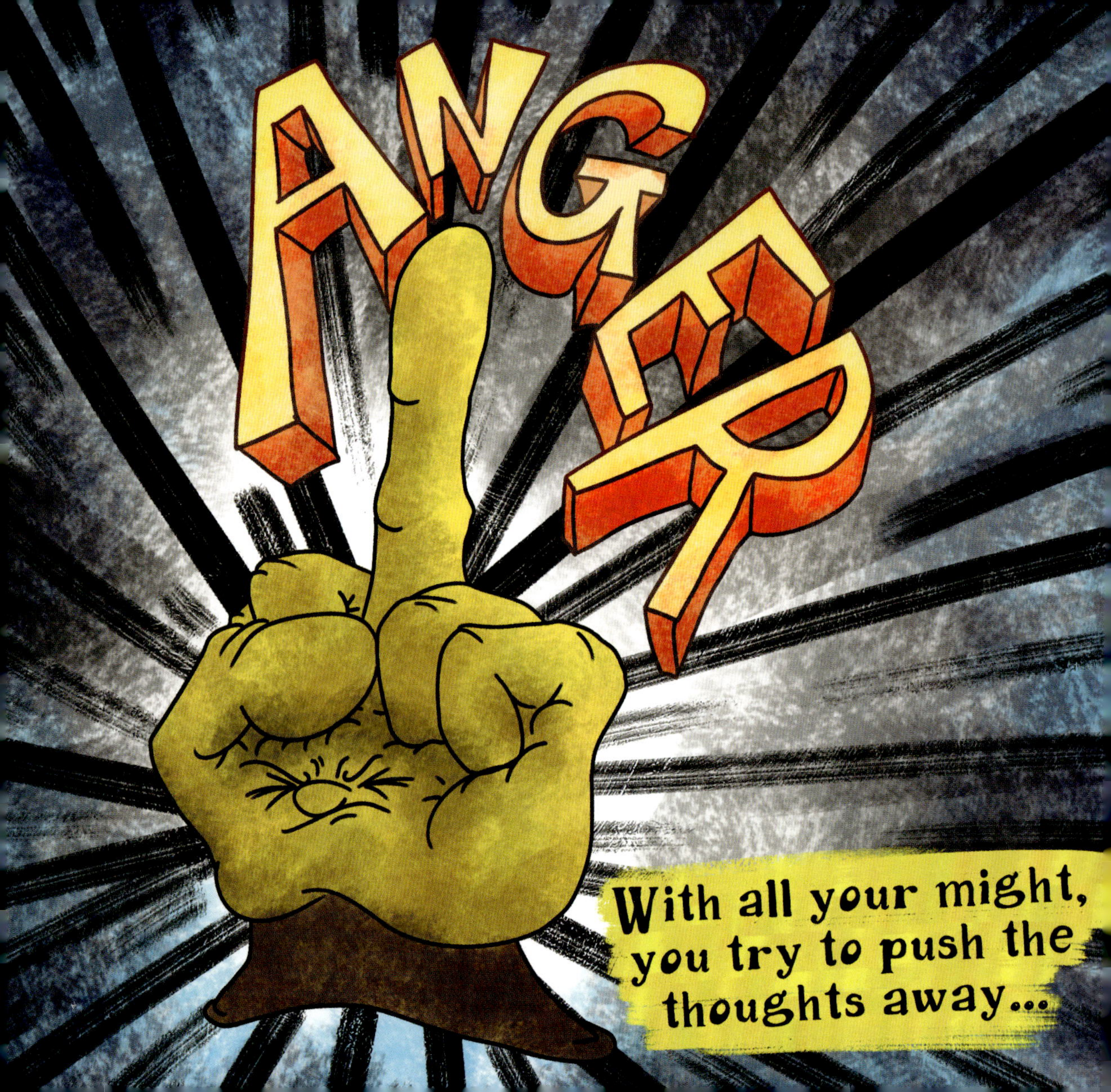
ANGER
With all your might, you try to push the thoughts away...

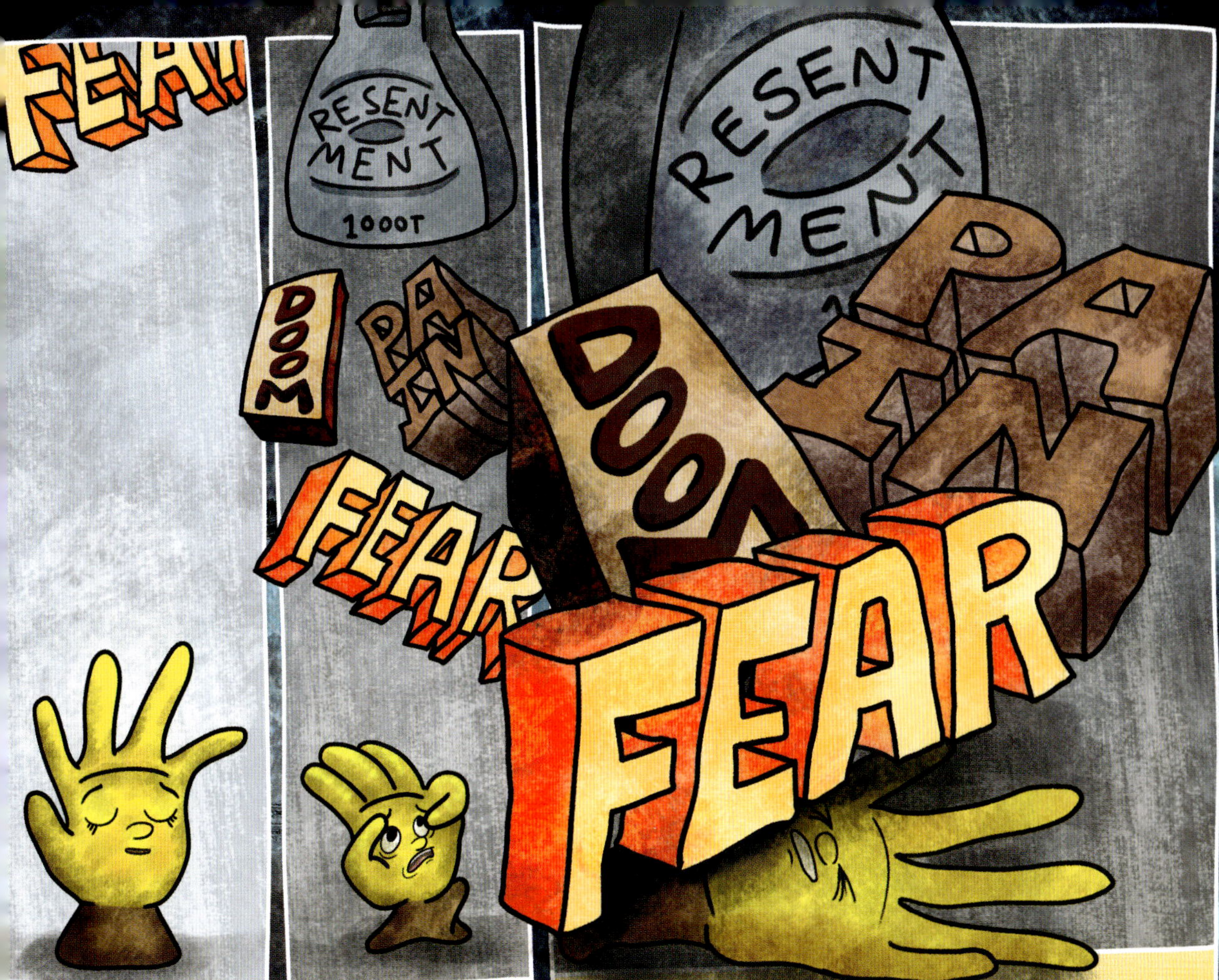

You might steal a moment to catch a breath ...

yet they just come back bigger, stronger

and cause more pain.

It's exhausting doing this every day, and you are running out of options.

It *is* exhausting.
I'm so **tired.**

Thinking about another hour of this pain **fills me with dread.**

I'm scared of what will happen if I have to live the rest of my life like this.

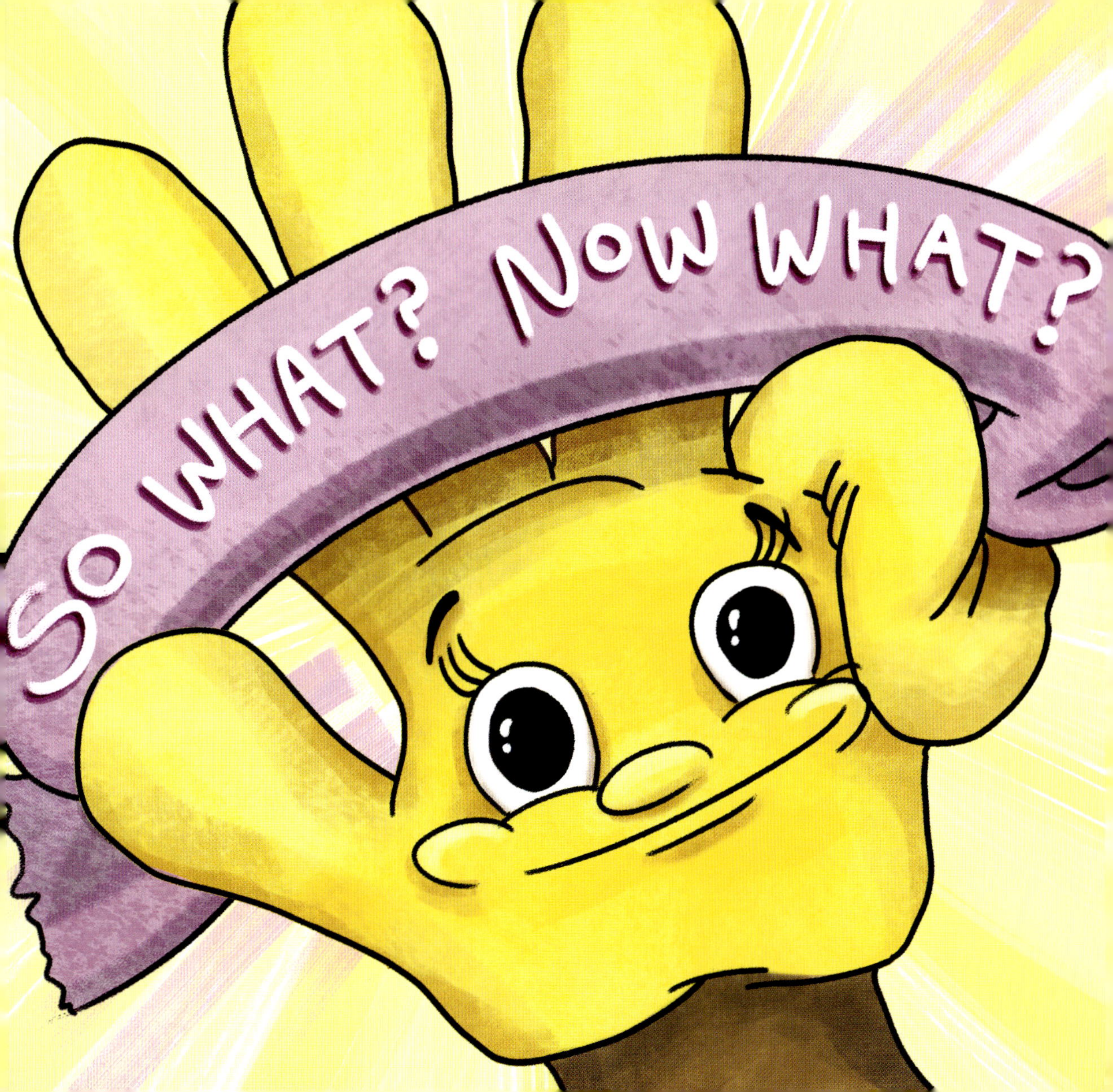
So WHAT? NoW WHAT?

What did you say?

I just told you that things are **so grim right now.** My ideas about making the **pain stop** are starting to involve ***some pretty permanent solutions.***

Yes, I heard you. That must be **really** awful. **So What? Now What?**

How can you walk and talk if you **don't have a heart?**

Oh but I do! I'm asking this because they're *questions* that helped me out of the same situation.

To ask **So What?** is to wholly accept what's beyond our control.

To ask **Now What?** is to push us into action, away from a place of pain.

Let me try another way...

Would it be fair to say that **everything** you've tried up to this point has felt like the **best idea at the time**?

Exactly.
I'm trying so hard.

I can see that.
I can also see that the best ideas you've chosen have landed you somewhere you don't want to be, and that you don't want to end up where you're heading.
What would happen if you tried out some *other ideas*?

I don't think **anything** will change.
Everything happens to me.
Always.
I have **no power** over where my life is heading.

So What? Now What?

Why do you keep saying that?

You're ignoring how **bad** this is for me.

So What? Now What?

If you weren't a **fictional cartoon character** I'd give you a ***"now what".***

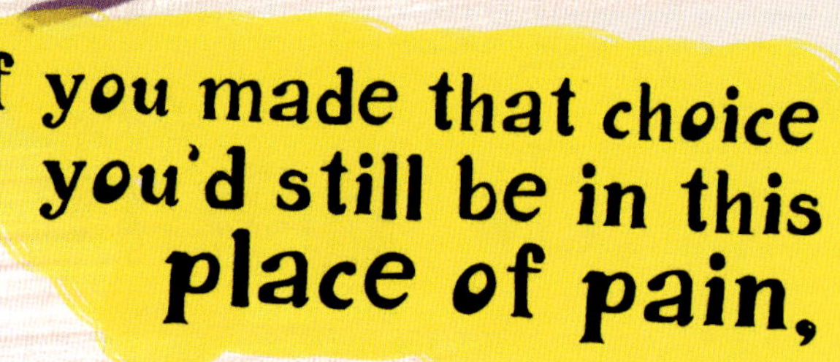

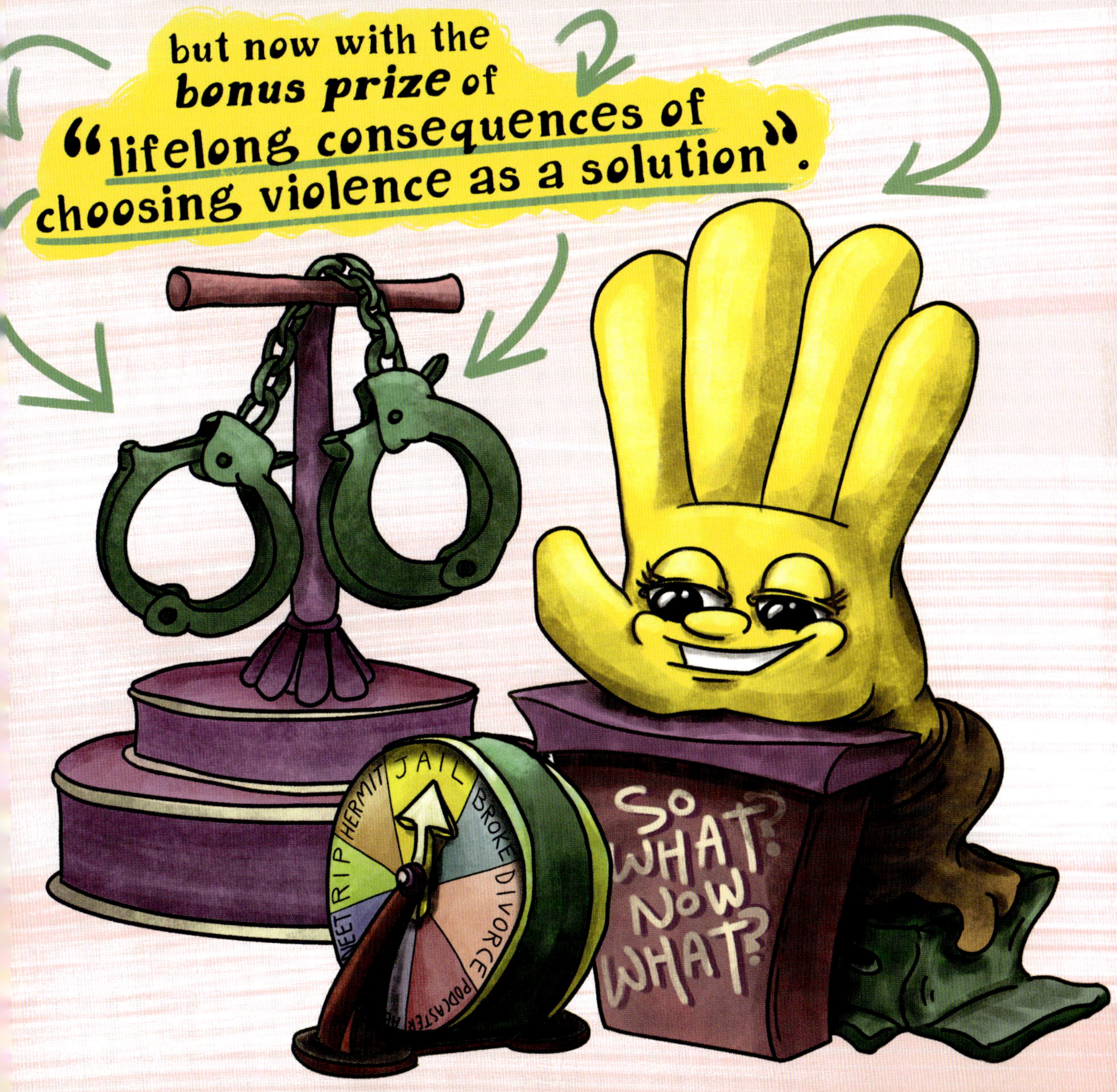
but now with the *bonus prize* of "lifelong consequences of choosing violence as a solution".
HERMIT
JAIL
BROKE
DIVORCE
PODCASTER
RIP
SO WHAT? NOW WHAT?

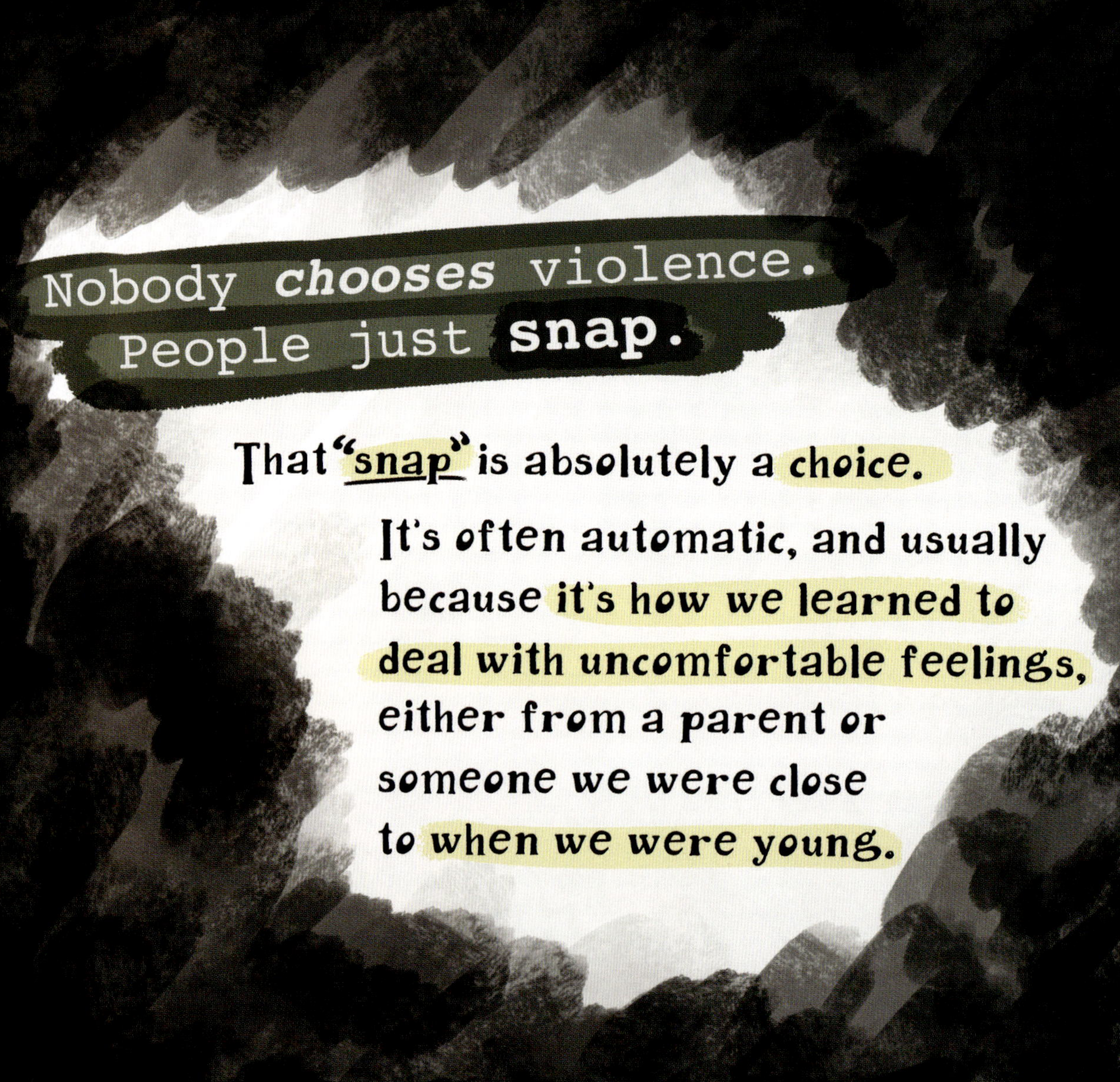
Nobody *chooses* violence.
People just **snap.**
That "snap" is absolutely a choice.
It's often automatic, and usually because it's how we learned to deal with uncomfortable feelings, either from a parent or someone we were close to when we were young.

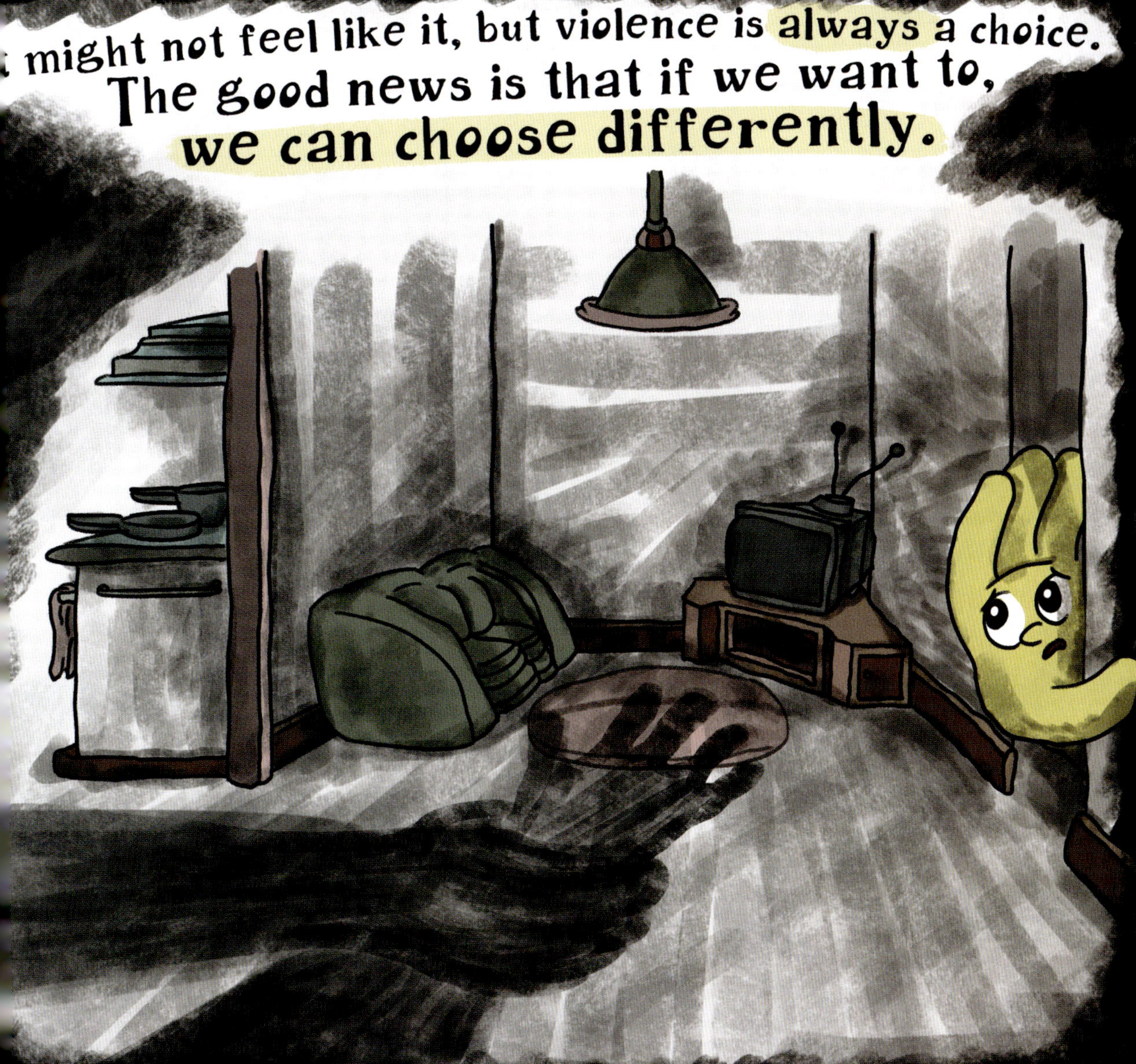
might not feel like it, but violence is always a choice.
The good news is that if we want to,
we can choose differently.

So if I want to feel any better
I have to make the ***choice*** to do so?

BINGO. Two choices actually.
There's the choice to say "So What?"
and then the choice to say "Now What?"

Nobody just "***chooses***" to feel better.
You're out of your mind.
Anyone in my situation
would feel the same.

You don't have to *like* what's happening.
However,
if you want things to feel better,
choosing to accept what's
happening is the first step.

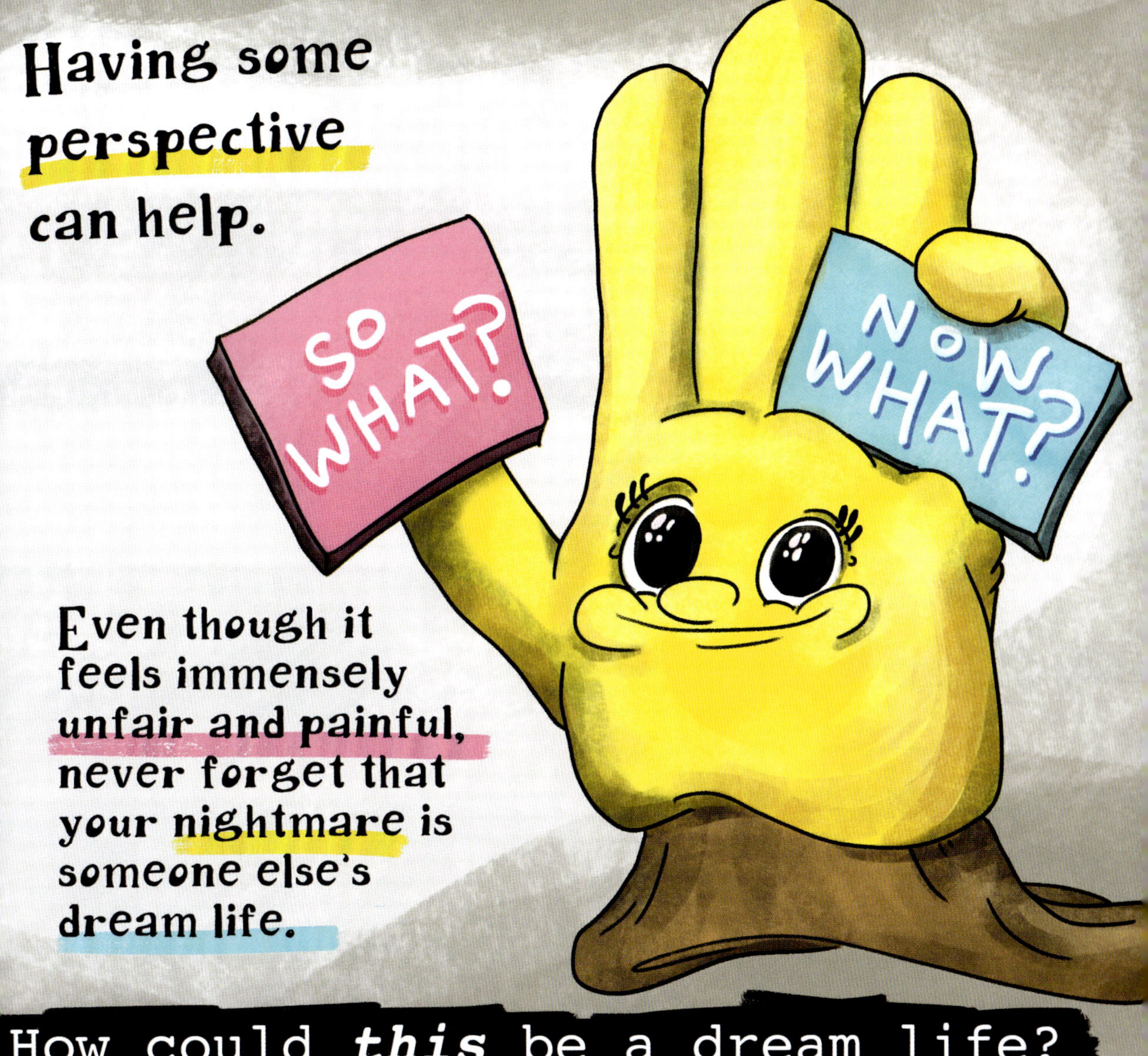
Having some perspective can help.
SO WHAT?
NOW WHAT?
Even though it feels immensely unfair and painful, never forget that your nightmare is someone else's dream life.
How could *this* be a dream life?

Do you know how to read?
Do you have time in your day to read?
Did you use a toilet today?
Did you drink water today that won't make you sick?
Are you reading this somewhere safe?

There are plenty of people who don't have one or more of those things, who would consider your situation an absolute dream.

Okay, so what about ***those people?***

You wouldn't tell a parent in a war zone trying to protect their kid from brutality and starvation *"So What? Now What?"*

This is all nonsense.

There's a version of this idea that was created out of a horrible situation just like that.

Viktor Frankl was an Austrian psychiatrist and psychotherapist.

Even though he lost his mother, father, brother and wife in the Holocaust, he survived years enduring the brutality of four concentration camps.

Noticing the differences between those prisoners who lived and those who died, he later wrote,

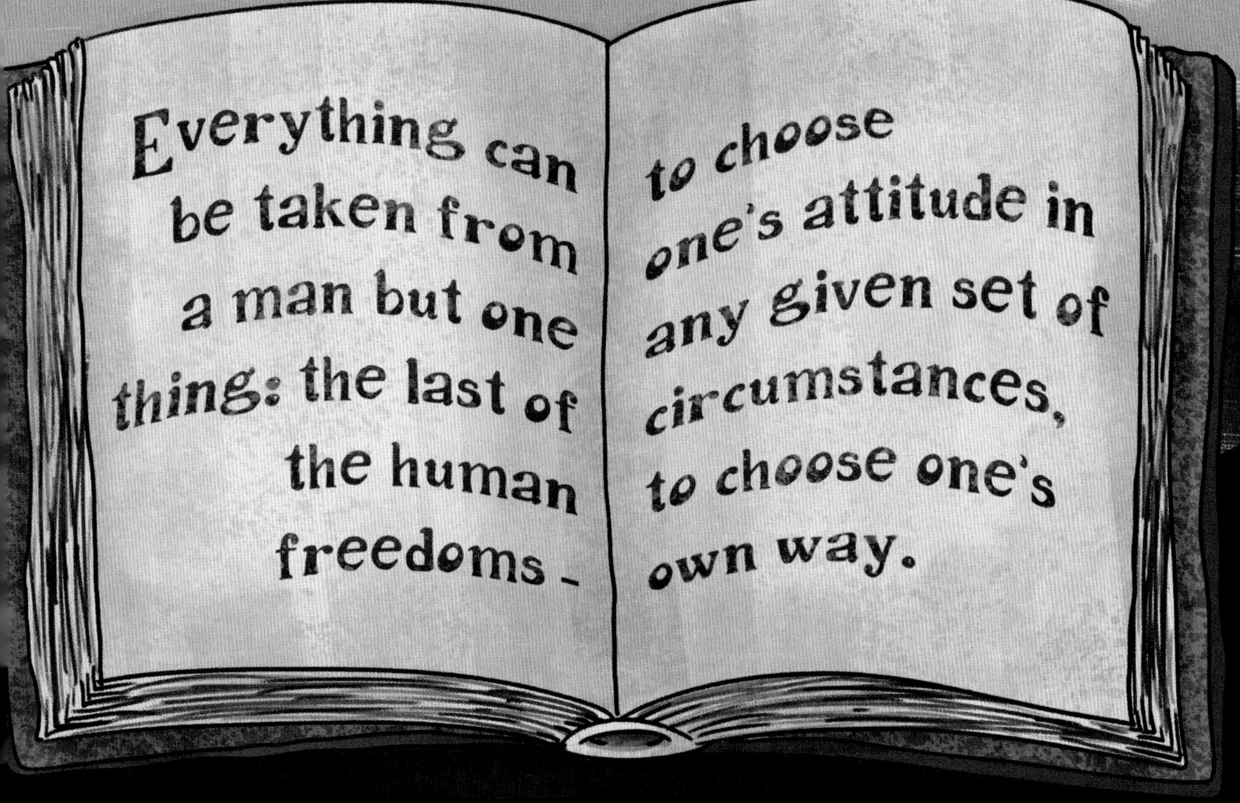

Everything can be taken from a man but one thing: the last of the human freedoms – to choose one's attitude in any given set of circumstances, to choose one's own way.

!!

So now you're making me feel guilty for complaining about my life.

I might not be in such an extreme situation, but there's so much I don't have, so much that's been taken from me.

And that must be tough.
I know you have at least one thing.

You still have the superpower possessed by all humans when they're born, yet so few know how to wield.

You have the ability to choose what you focus on, and what action you'll take.

You have had this *power* all along.

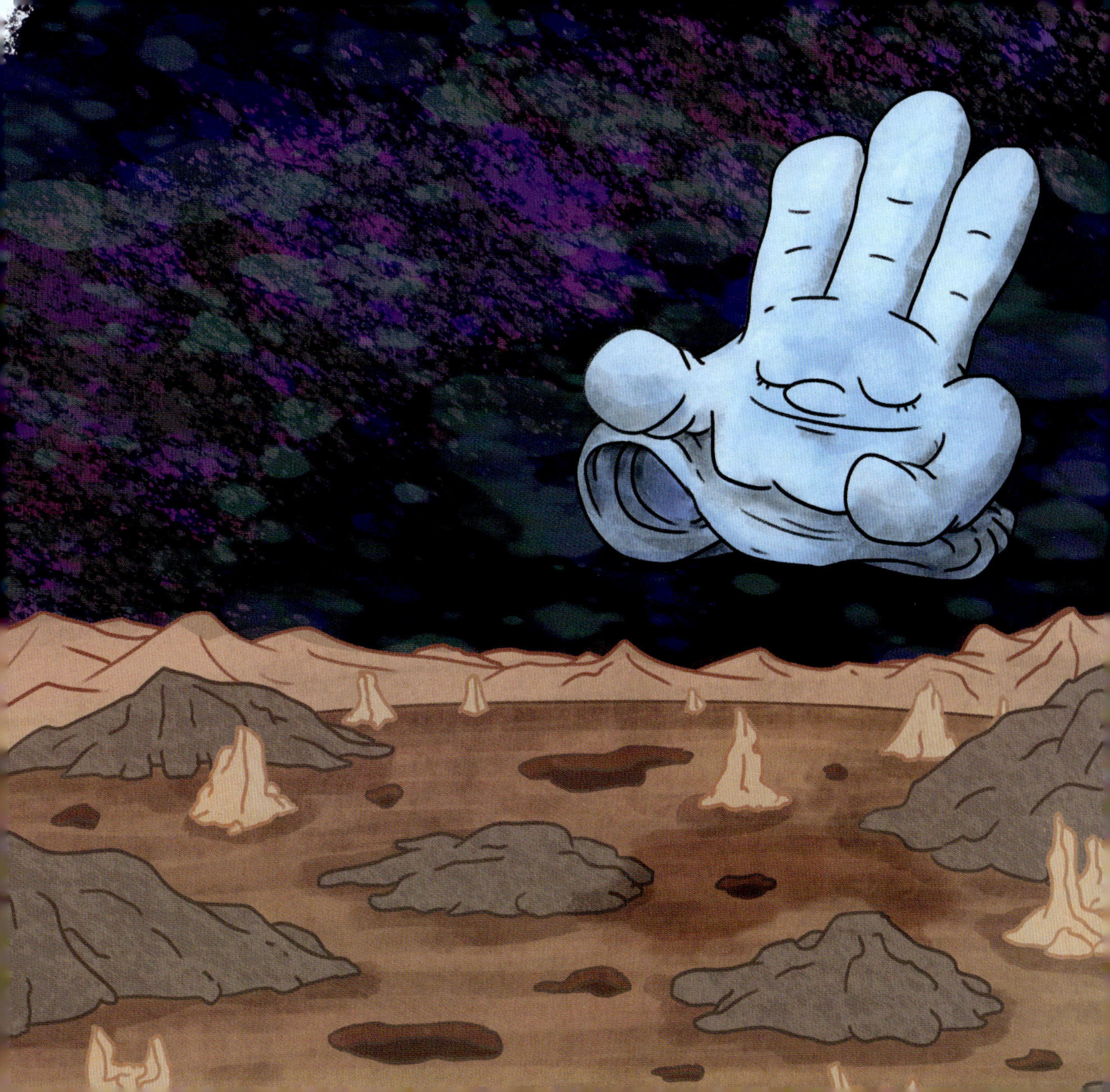

Would you knock it off?

This is like some **lame movie** where the **wizard** shows up at **the end** and tells the hero,

"Oh my child, but you've always been special!"

You're not about to do that, are you?

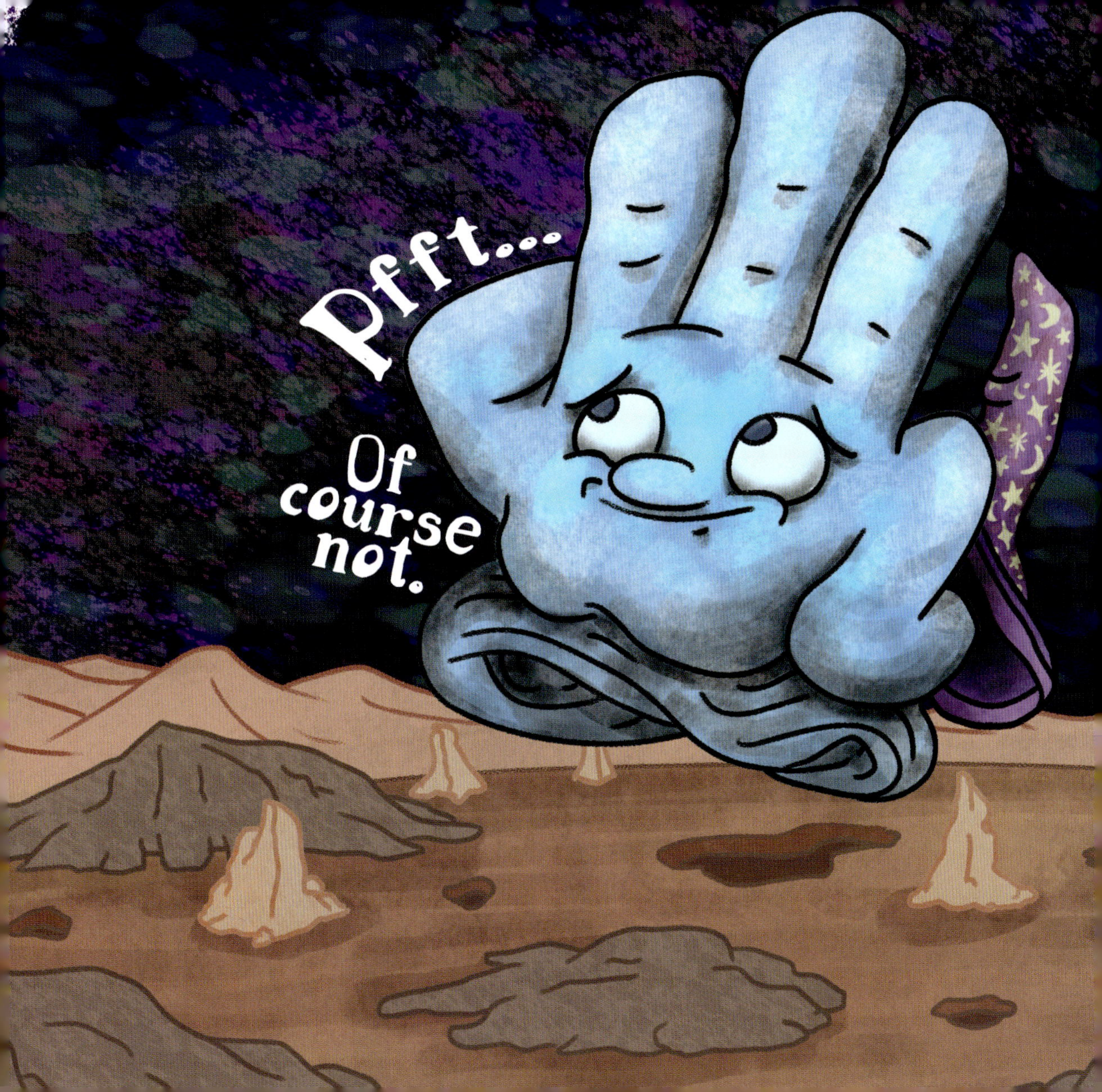
Pffft...
Of course not.

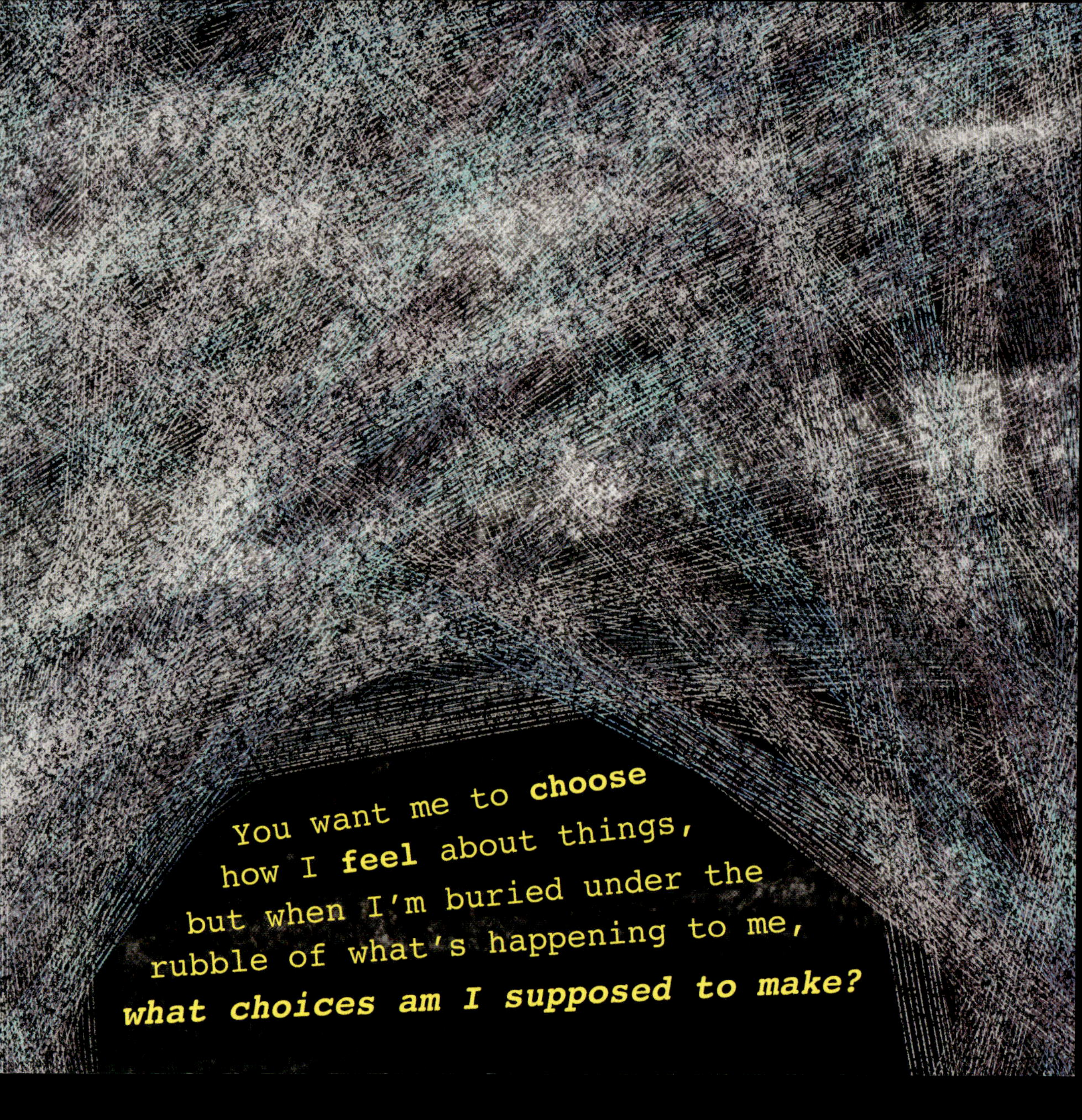
You want me to **choose**
how I **feel** about things,
but when I'm buried under the
rubble of what's happening to me,
what choices am I supposed to make?

Try starting with "So What?"

Choose to fully accept that most of life is completely out of our control, and it's nothing but fantasy to wish for any of it to be different.

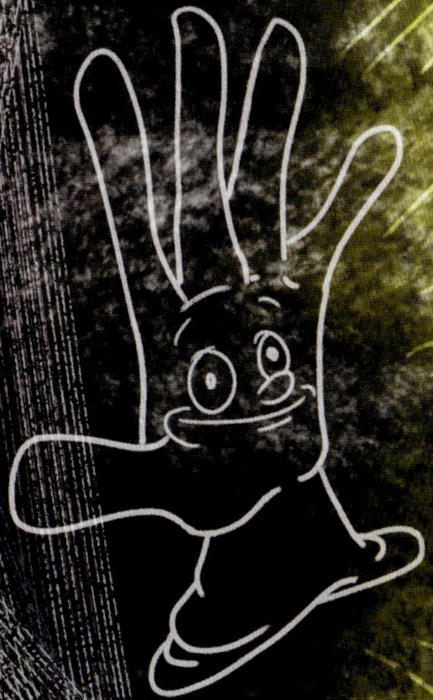

And considering that sometimes the only way out of the flames is through them, we need to get moving.

The choice of "Now What?" is to deliberately and actively move towards a goal we value.

Remember: it's not about the size of the stride, it's about the motivation to keep moving.

Now you're just repeating things you learned from a fortune cookie.

-MENU-
SADNESS
SADNESS with Rice
SADNESS (steamed)
SADNESS SALAD
with salty tears
vinaigrette

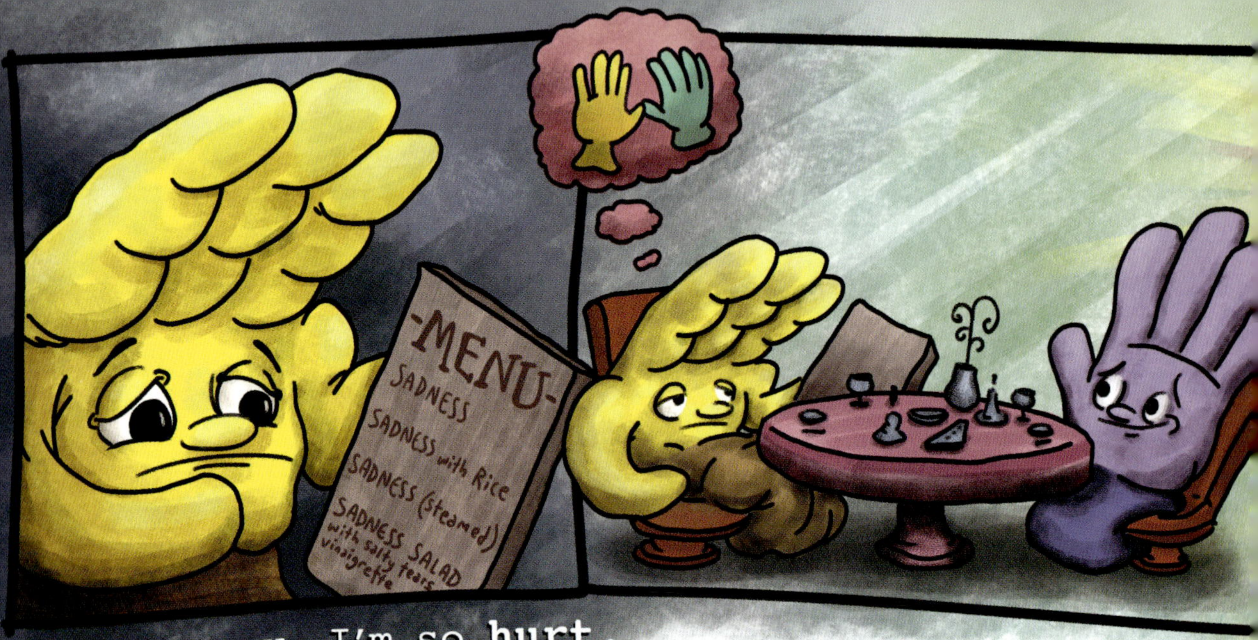

I'm so **angry**. I'm so **hurt**.

I don't want to accept some of the things that are happening to me.

I just can't make that choice.

Choosing not to accept that a relationship is over can keep you sitting in sadness, instead of going out and meeting someone else, or worse: sabotagin any new relationship you get into.

Then recognise that as long as you choose to **resist acceptance**, all those other things will make your choices for you.

Your ex has already moved o

You're choosing to give them control over your ability to find happiness.

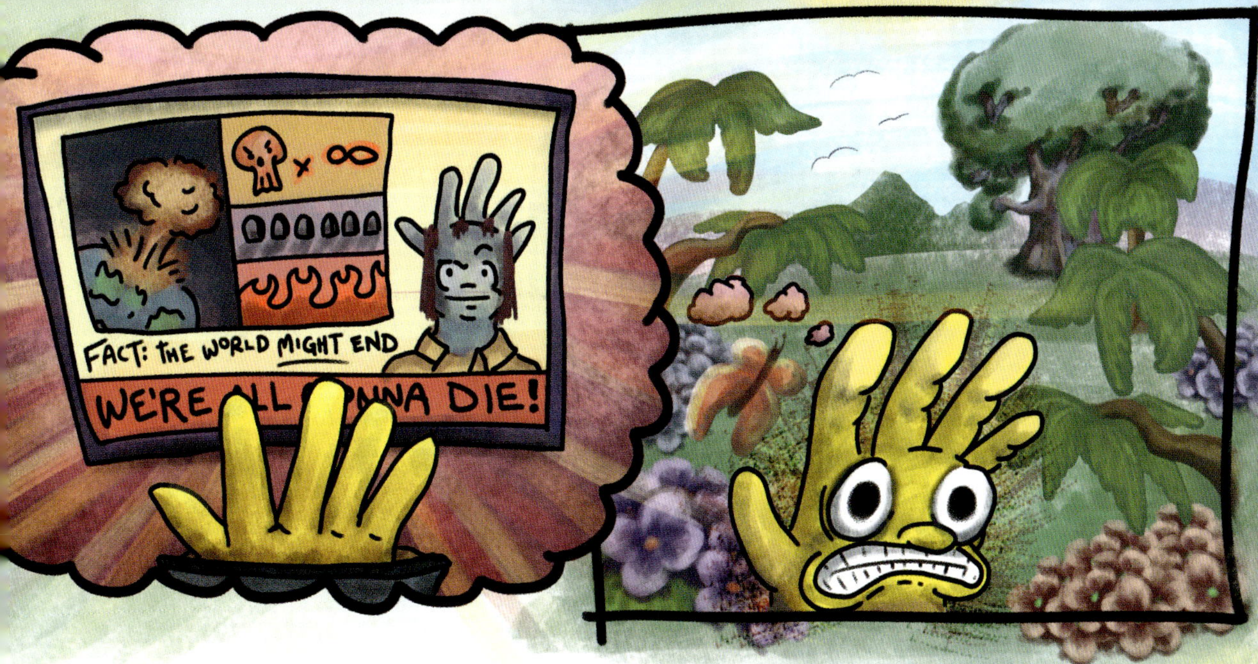

f you're worried about a global conflict in the news, you won't hear the birds singing, smell the flowers or enjoy the warmth of the sun on your skin.

The news doesn't care about your feelings; you're choosing to let it prevent you from feeling joy.

Refusing to accept things as they are takes away our control over our lives.

It robs us of happiness.

But it's all **so overwhelming.** The **smallest thing** related to any of the pain I'm in causes a **huge reaction** in me.

Of course it does. That's what your brain is designed to do.

Sounds like a pretty useless design to me.

Our brains can sometimes make life difficult, but it's important to understand that your brain and body are identical to humans known to have lived at least 300,000 years ago.

The dangerous world we evolved to live in no longer exists, yet there are parts of our brain that still react to threat, or the idea of threat, as if we're face to face with a Quinkana – the seven-metre-long land crocodile with massive legs that lived in Australia until only 10,000 years ago – or one of those giant eagles in Africa that was so big it could literally pick up a child by the skull and fly off.

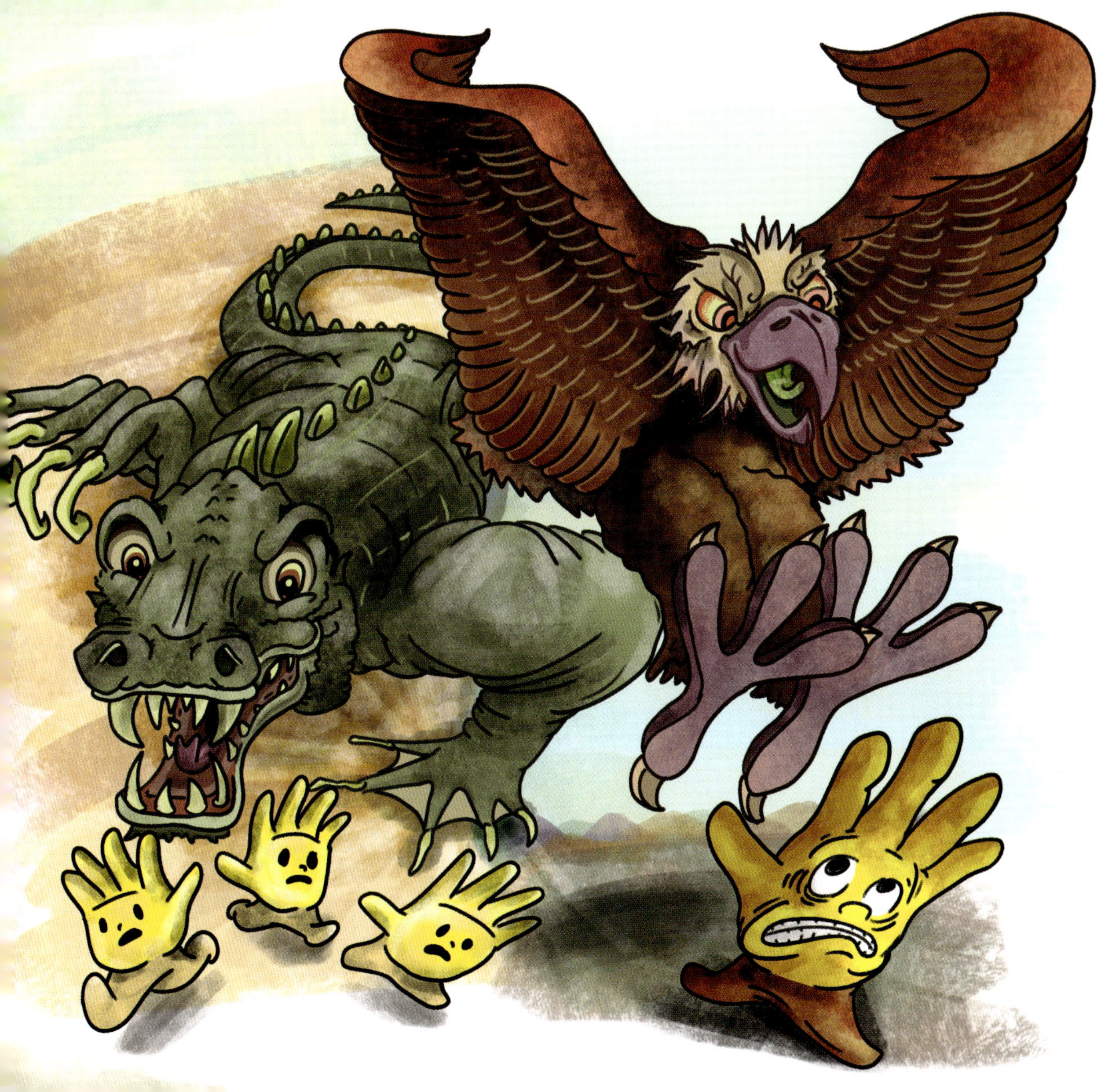

That's terrifying.

Exactly.

And you've evolved to think that.

We're only alive because you and me and everyone we know are the descendants of people who saw the

RAPIDLY GROWING SHADOW

below them and ran away.

The ones who got excited and said, "Oooh, Birdy!", didn't make it.

Seeing a shadow set off their "fight-or-flight" response, flooding their body with stress hormones and giving them the surge of energy to escape.

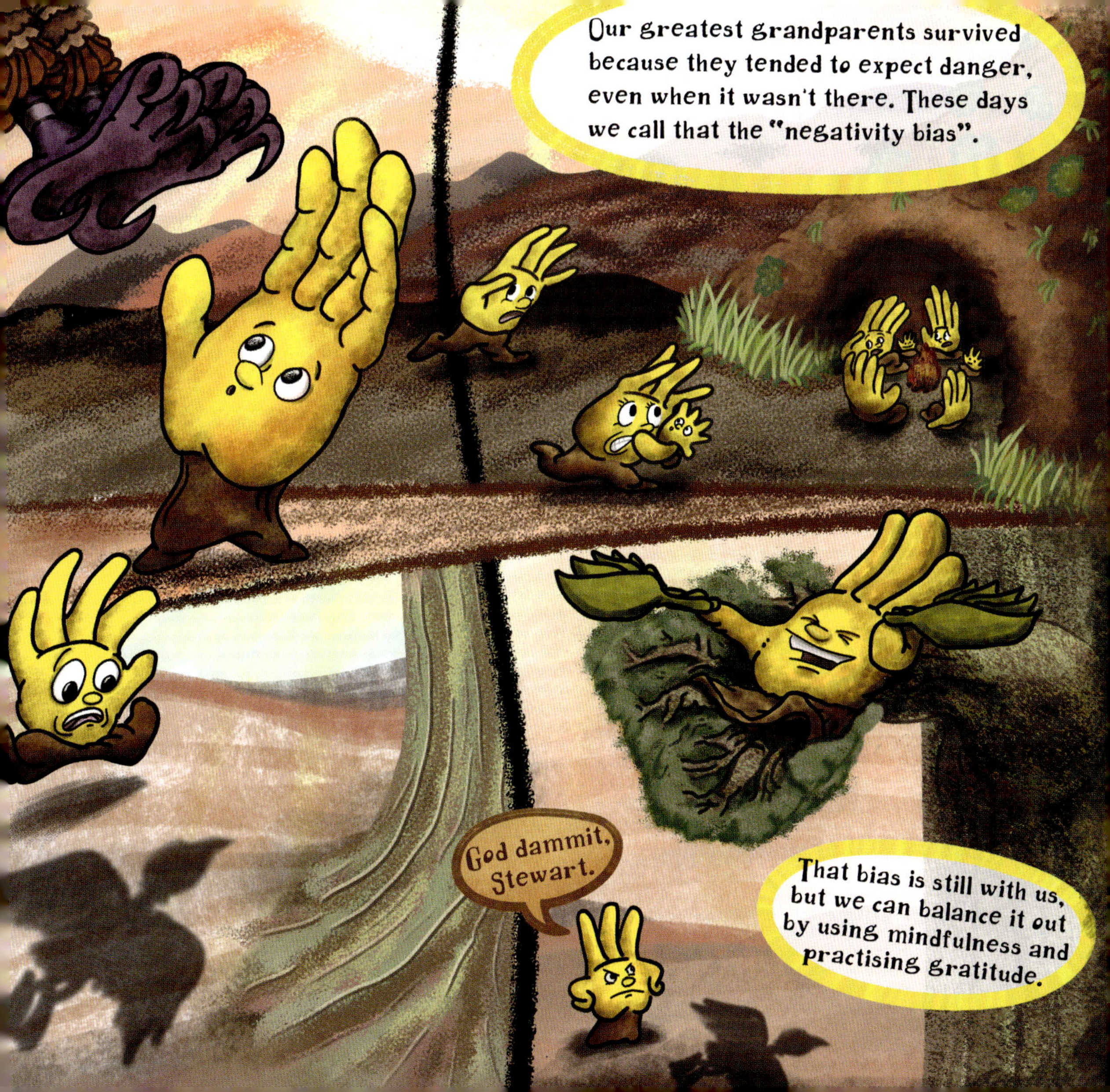
Our greatest grandparents survived because they tended to expect danger, even when it wasn't there. These days we call that the "negativity bias".
God dammit, Stewart.
That bias is still with us, but we can balance it out by using mindfulness and practising gratitude.

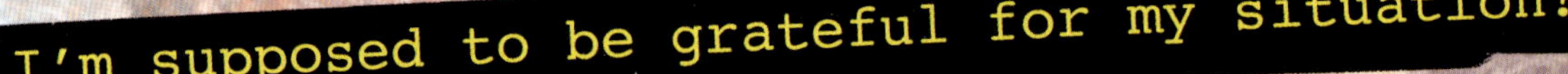

You're unbelievable.

It's one of the ways to keep a balanced view on our experience.

And it starts with noticing times when you got lucky.

What, like winning the lotto?

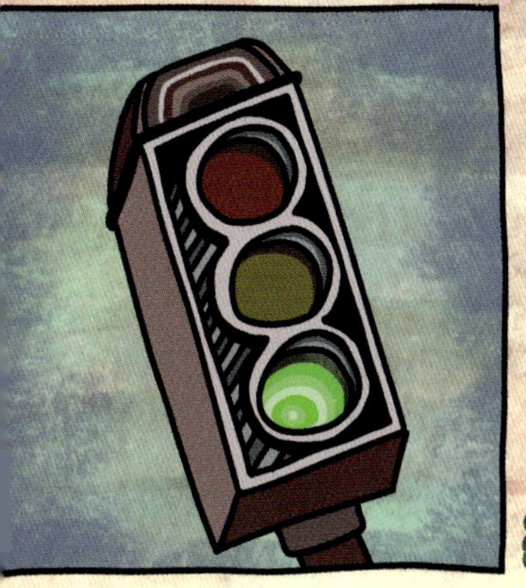

More like noticing when you caught a green light,

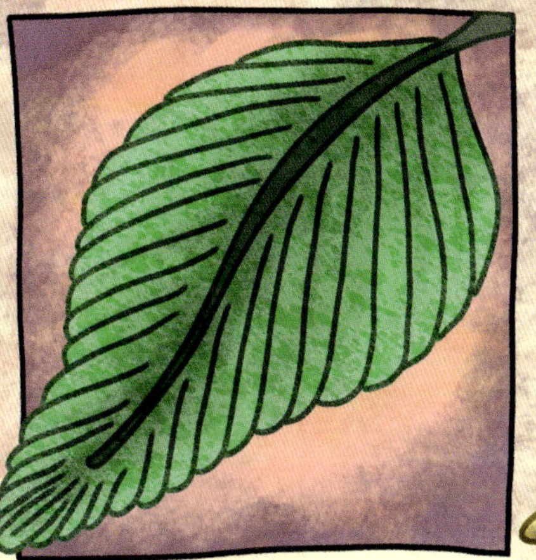

glimpsed a fleeting moment of beauty in nature,

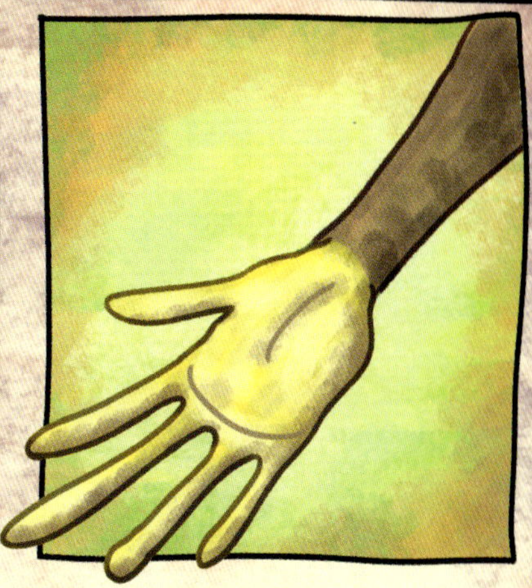

or was in the right place when someone needed a hand.

Look for three things every day, tell someone you care about or write them down.

The more we notice when things go well, the more we notice when things go well.

Over time, our experience of life changes.

I don't think I'd notice any difference.

Well, that brings us to mindfulness ...

Did you ever do a burpee in PE at school?

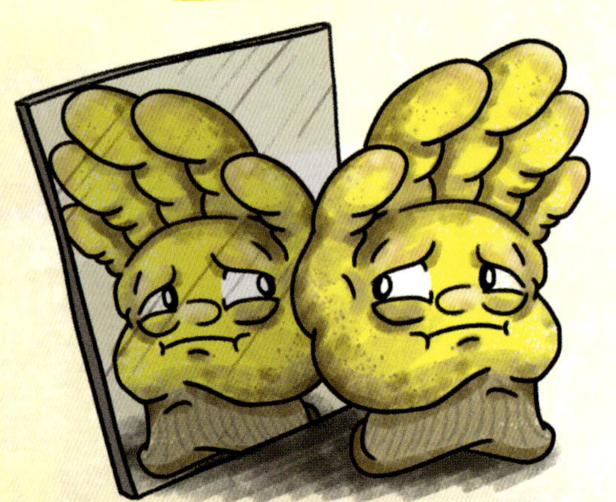

I just threw up in my mouth a bit even thinking about them.

Yeah, they're the worst.

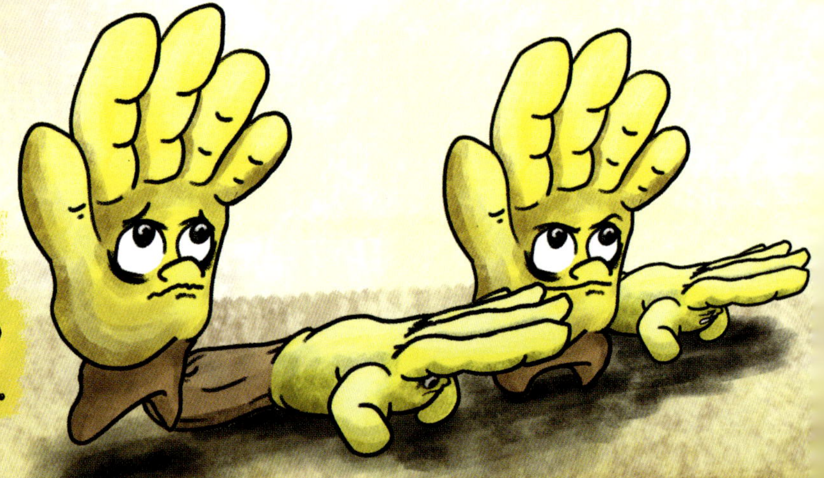

But burpees are possibly the best full-body strength and conditioning exercise you can do in a confined space.

100 burpees a day for 30 days will radically change your physical fitness.

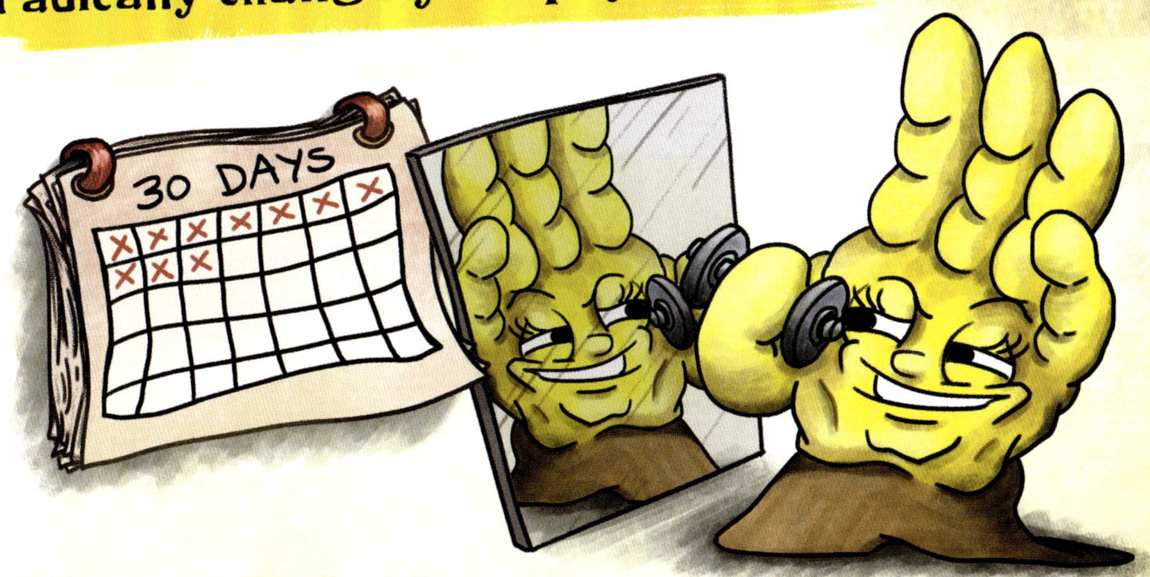

So what if I told you there was a burpee for the brain?

As long as I don't puke.

I doubt you'll puke; it's just noticing.

You already know how to do it, because you've described that you think about your thinking.

The Zen Buddhists describe this by identifying these two minds as the "thinking mind" and the "observing mind".

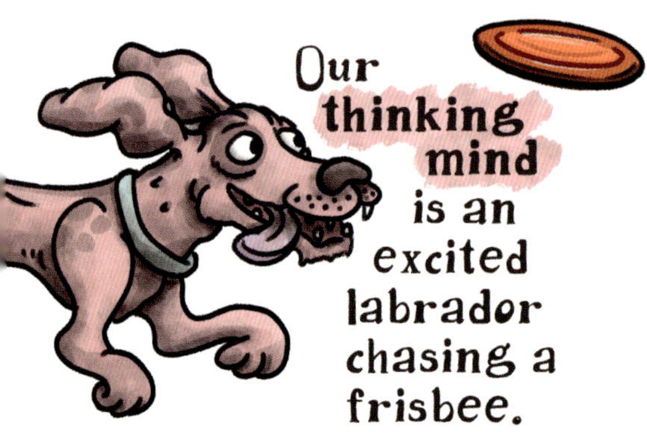

Our **thinking mind** is an excited labrador chasing a frisbee.

Our **observing mind** is sitting on a park bench watching that labrador about to joyfully run straight onto a busy freeway.

Yet if the **labrador** runs onto the freeway, the **observing mind** also feels the consequences.

When we're flooded with emotion, we can get stuck in "thinking mind", and it's almost impossible to choose anything but chasing the frisbee.

To give us other choices, we need to build up the strength of the "observing mind".

A simple way to start is by **breathing and noticing.**

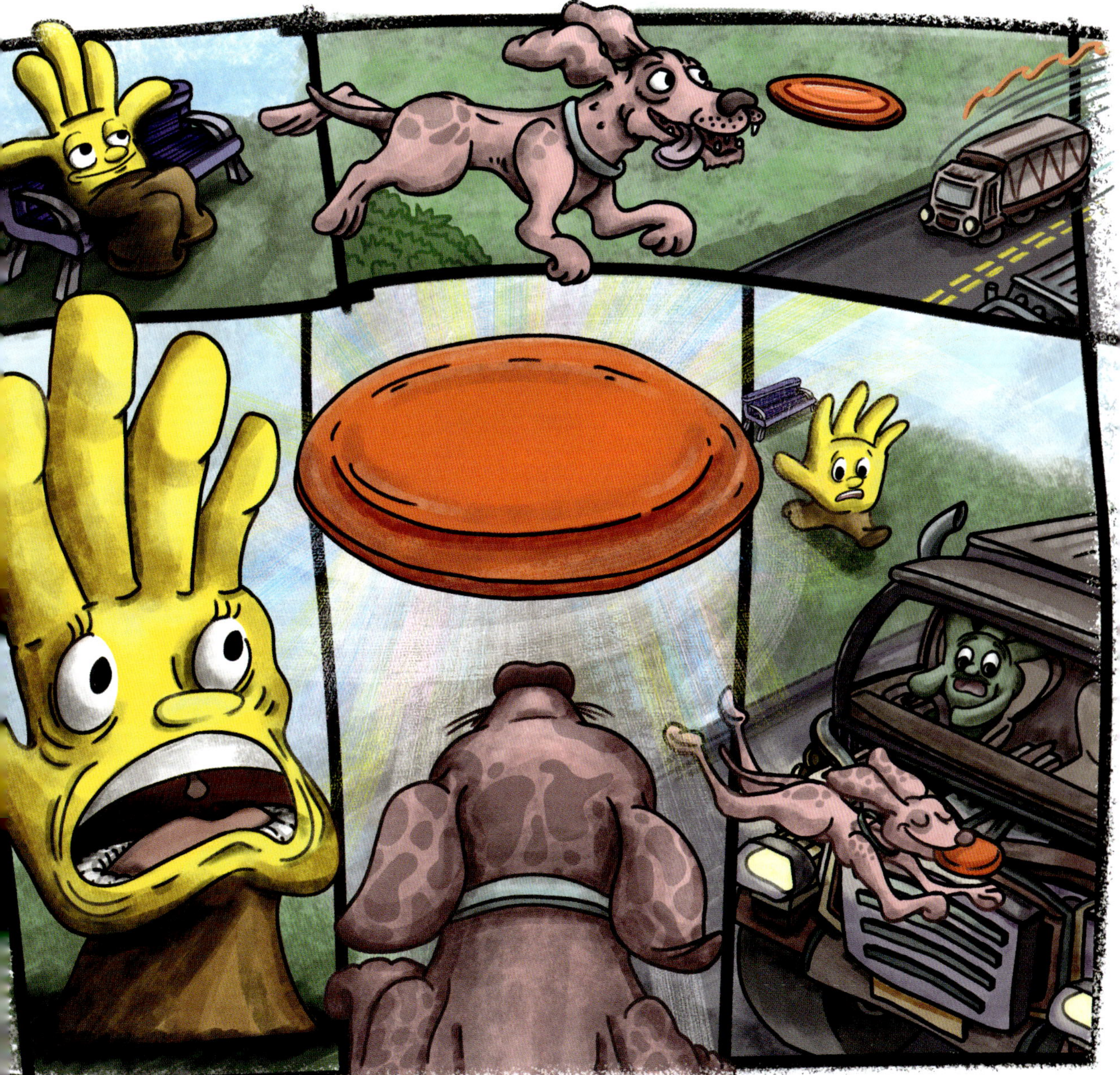

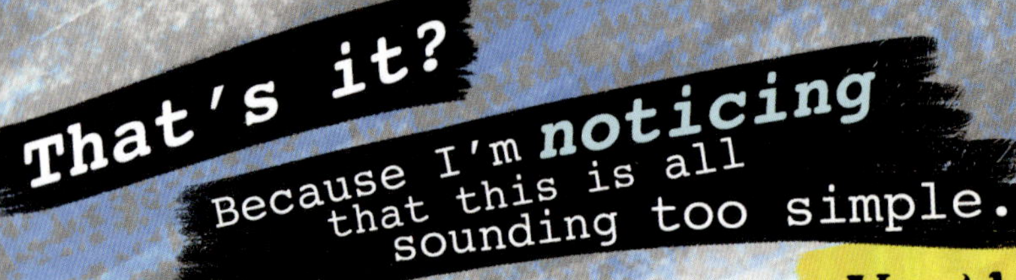

You'd be surprised.

It can be tricky.

To start with, try putting the words "I'm noticing" in front of a physical feeling.

I'm noticing the weight of this book.

I'm noticing the position my body is in.

Notice your breath.

What happens when you slow your breathing down?

Notice what emotions you're feeling.

Noticing helps the observing mind get used to jumping into emotionally intense moments to take a look over things, and hopefully give us more **choices.**

There you go *again* about ***choices.***

When are you going to understand that I didn't ***choose*** *any of this* to happen to me?

True.
However, whether you realise it or not, you're choosing how you feel about it.
As humans, we choose our entire reality. It's what we do.

When you see the Southern Cross in the night sky,

what's actually happening is photons

which have travelled quadrillions of kilometres through space, across hundreds of light years

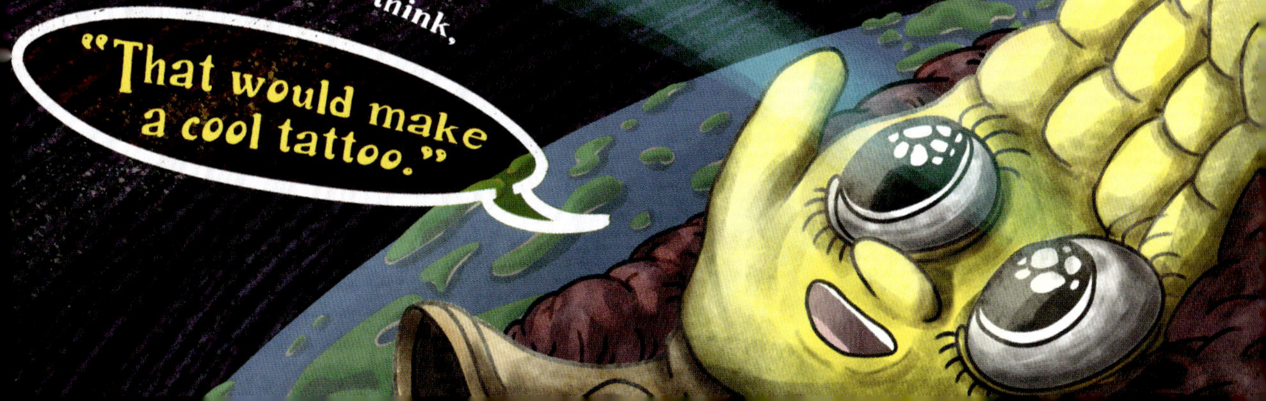

Yet neither the photon, nor that star, care if we call it the Southern Cross.

We only have names for anything because as humans we make stuff mean stuff.

And when our brains are healthy, we can notice the thoughts that we have about stuff.

It's okay if they're uncomfortable thoughts - we can make some room for them and then take a step towards what we value.

are hitting your eyeball, only for your brain to think,

"That would make a cool tattoo."

Okay, Neil DeGlove Tyson, how can I **choose** to make what's happening to me mean **anything other than something terrible?**

By choosing to accept what's happening to you, and then choosing what you do next.

What do you mean?
How am I supposed to know what to do next?

Easy.
Choose to take action in accordance with your values.

Values again!
What is that supposed to mean?

Each of us has our own set of values.
What we value in ourselves, our families, our friends and the society we live in.

What's happening to me feels **very unfair.**
Do I *value* **fairness?**

Yes, "fairness" or "justice" is a widely held value of modern society.

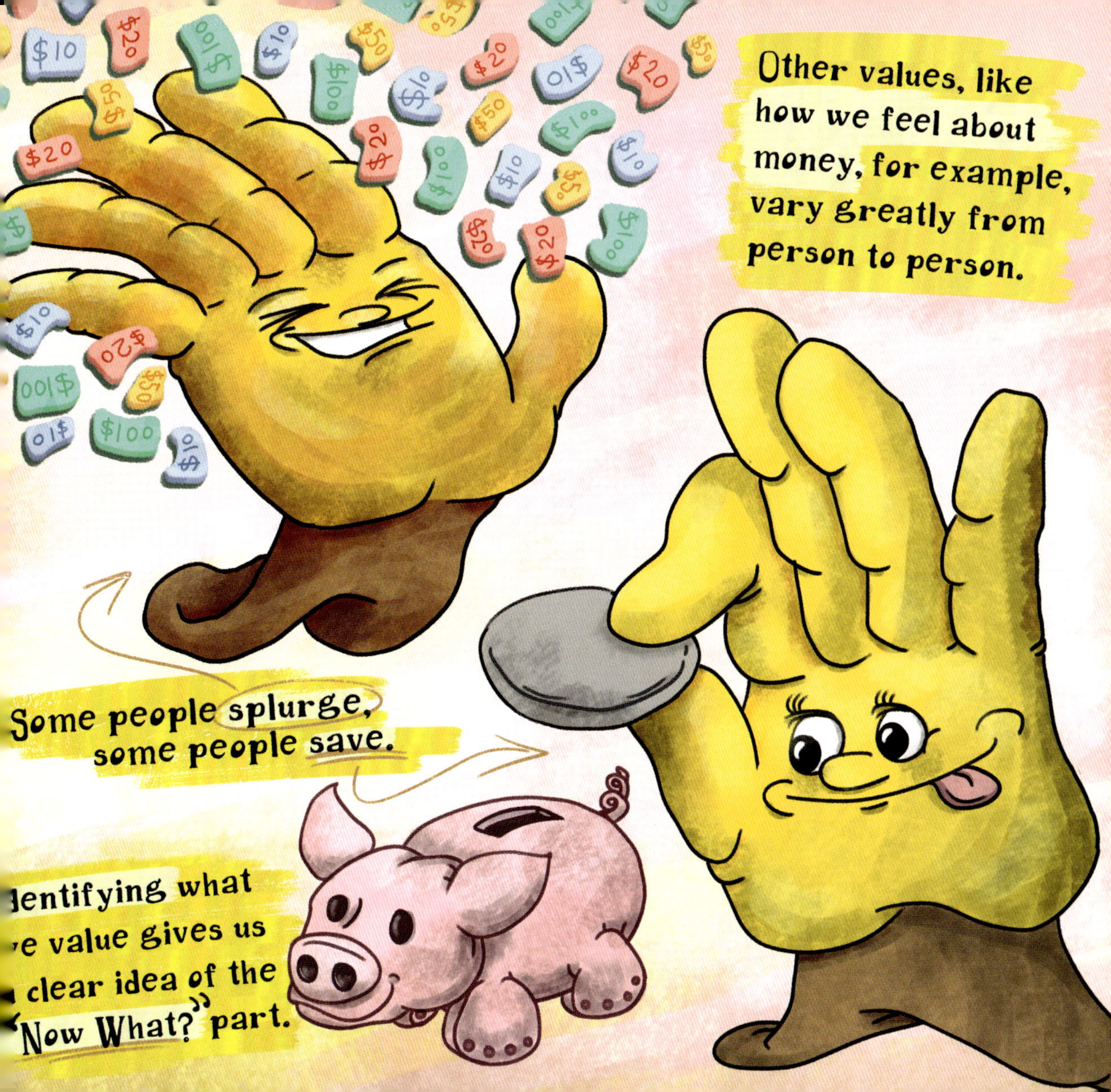
Other values, like how we feel about money, for example, vary greatly from person to person.
Some people splurge, some people save.
dentifying what
e value gives us
clear idea of the
'Now What?" part.

So if I hurt because
I don't feel any compassion
or kindness from my friends,
those are probably values too.

How can I move towards compassion or kindness without them?

You could start with having compassion and kindness for yourself.

When we've been doing it tough for a while,
after enough time feeling bad
even though we've
been doing our best,
sometimes we make ourselves feel worse
because we're not "better" yet.

One way to move towards the goal of feeling differently
is to consider some kindness and compassion
for those you feel have wronged you.

You want me to forgive them?

Acceptance of others
doesn't mean
forgiveness of others,
if you're not ready for that.

Trying to understand their motivations
can go a long way to making things feel better.

You're doing the best you can
with the best ideas you have right now.

So is everyone else.

Each of us bears a responsibility for
the impact our choices have on others,
and ...

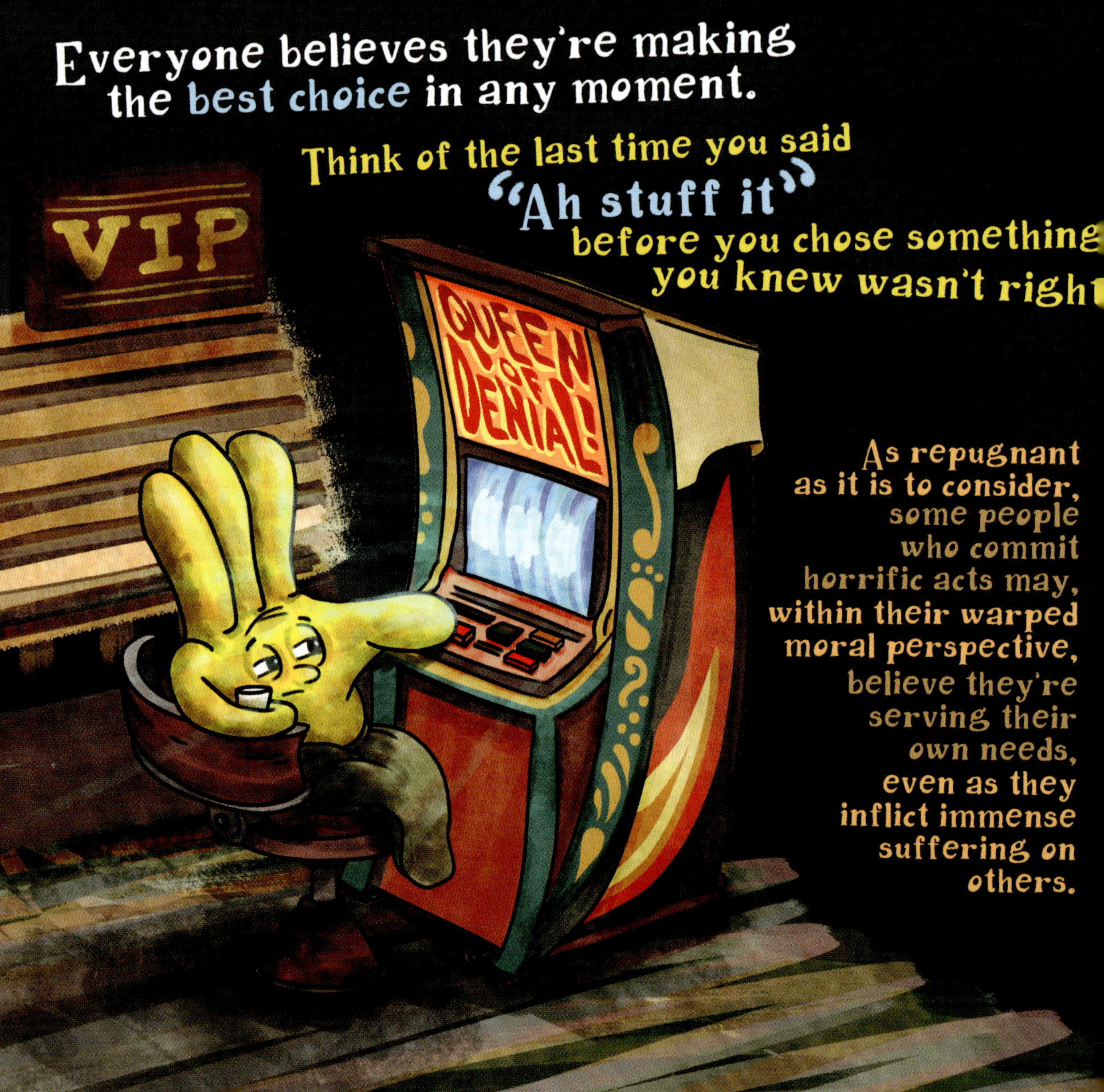

Everyone believes they're making the best choice in any moment.
Think of the last time you said "Ah stuff it" before you chose something you knew wasn't right
VIP
QUEEN OF DENIAL!
As repugnant as it is to consider, some people who commit horrific acts may, within their warped moral perspective, believe they're serving their own needs, even as they inflict immense suffering on others.

That's really hard to think about.

I don't know if I can do it.

Yeah, it is hard, and it does take work. And you'll probably avoid doing that work for as long as you possibly can.

But sooner or later *the fear* of doing that work becomes less than *the pain* of staying the same.

Nothing changes unless we change.

So you're asking me to **accept pain,**
accept heartache and **accept loss**
if I want **any chance of happiness?**

*That doesn't make **sense!***

Do you value **courage?**

Of course.

If you have the courage to do those burpees we all dislike so much, to willingly experience the discomfort of the work, your body will adapt by growing more muscle, improving your fitness and giving you greater physical resilience and flexibility.

Having the courage to be with uncomfortable thoughts and feelings builds our emotional resilience.

It gives us the confidence to make bold choices, and we're rewarded with a rich life, full of meaning.

But sometimes the thoughts and feelings aren't just **uncomfortable**, they're ***unbearable***.

They start to cascade out of control.

I'll see or hear something that reminds me of why everything hurts and my whole body gets caught in a downward spiral that gets worse and worse.

When it's **really bad**, even the most harmless and unrelated things can **transport me back** to exactly how it felt in the middle of a **horrible moment** from my **past** or forward into a **terrifying imagined future**, as if it were happening **right now**.

It's like being sucked through the screen into a horror movie I never wanted to watch.

There's a name for that horrendous feeling of "being unable to escape because the pain is everywhere you turn."

When our thoughts are so powerful that we can no longer ignore them, when we treat our thoughts as absolute facts even if they're not real, when thoughts start to control our emotions and actions, that's called "cognitive fusion."

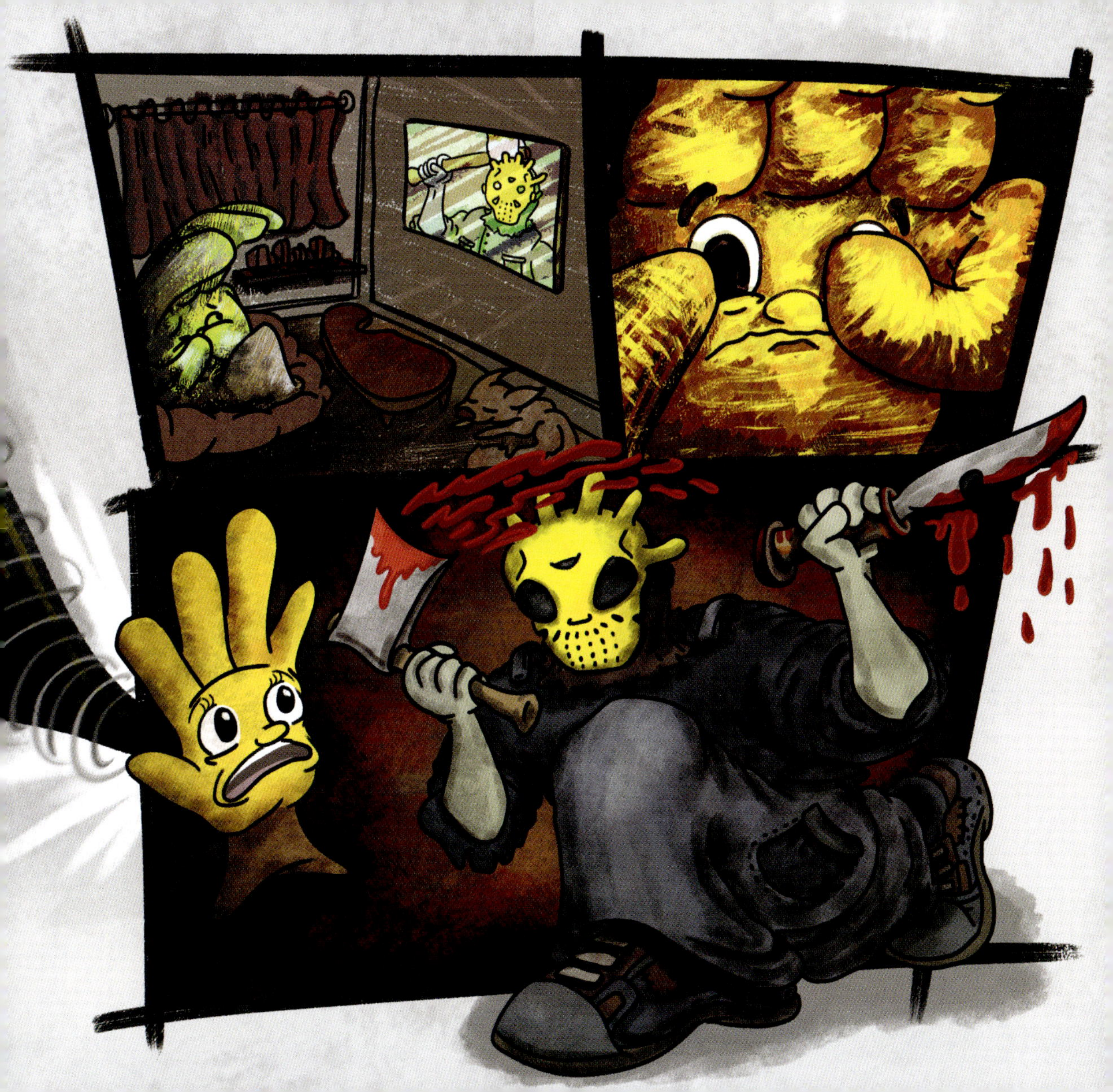

I don't see how asking "Now What?" could make a difference when I can **barely breathe.**

You're actually asking "Now What?" without realising it. You're noticing your breath, and you're noticing the thoughts.

That's a great start.

I notice the thoughts, then feel awful that they're still there. Even if I manage to avoid them through distraction or trying to push them away through unhealthy behaviours,

they come back even stronger.

It's futile.

Yeah, it can really feel pointless.

Your brain can falsely convince you that this is how things will be forever, which is a very dangerous place to be.

Why would our brains deliberately want to self-destruct like that?

When our survival instincts get out of balance, it can sometimes happen. Understanding those instincts is the key to escaping that trap.

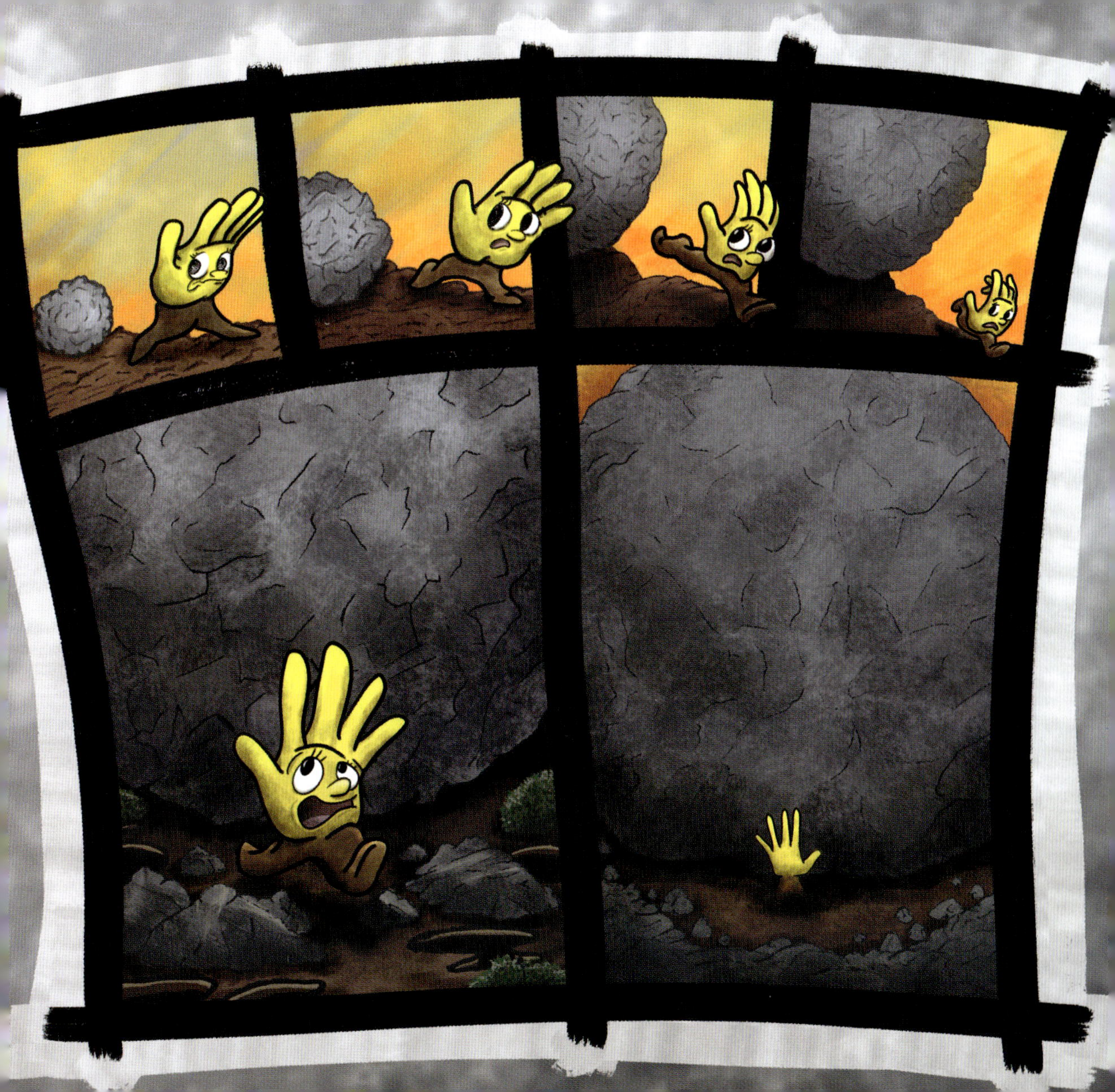

When *Thoughts and Feelings* are smothering you, it can feel like your thinking mind is in a **deep hole** with painful *Thoughts and Feelings* throwing dirt down the hole **one shovel at a time.**

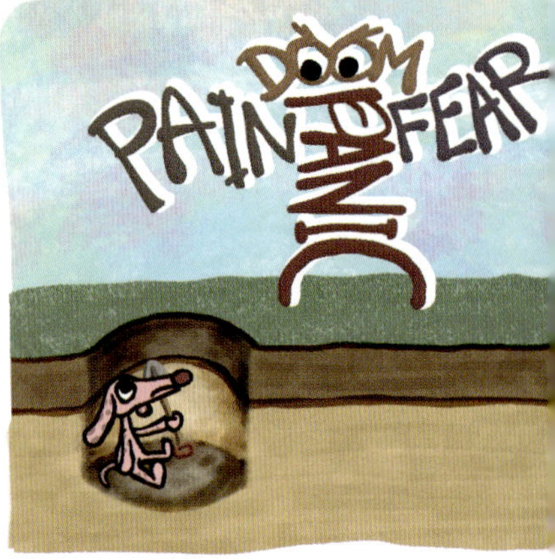

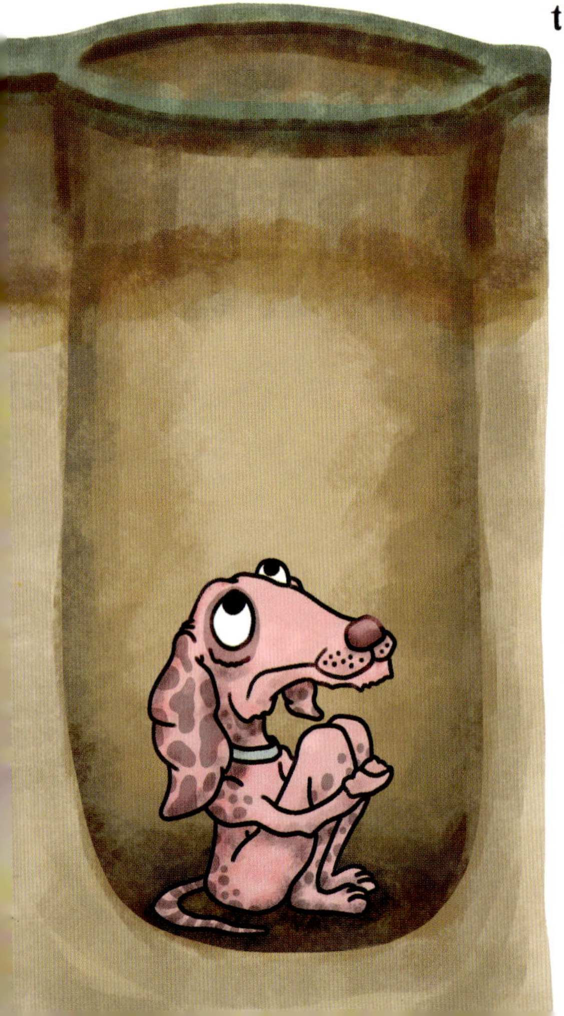

It's suffocating and you'll do *anything* to escape, so the thinking mind digs out **two shovels** of dirt for every **one** that pours down.

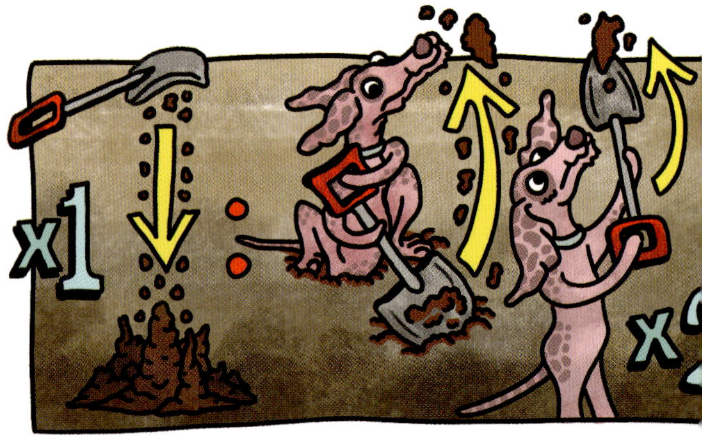

It may even be a relief to feel like you're doing something about the situation you're in.

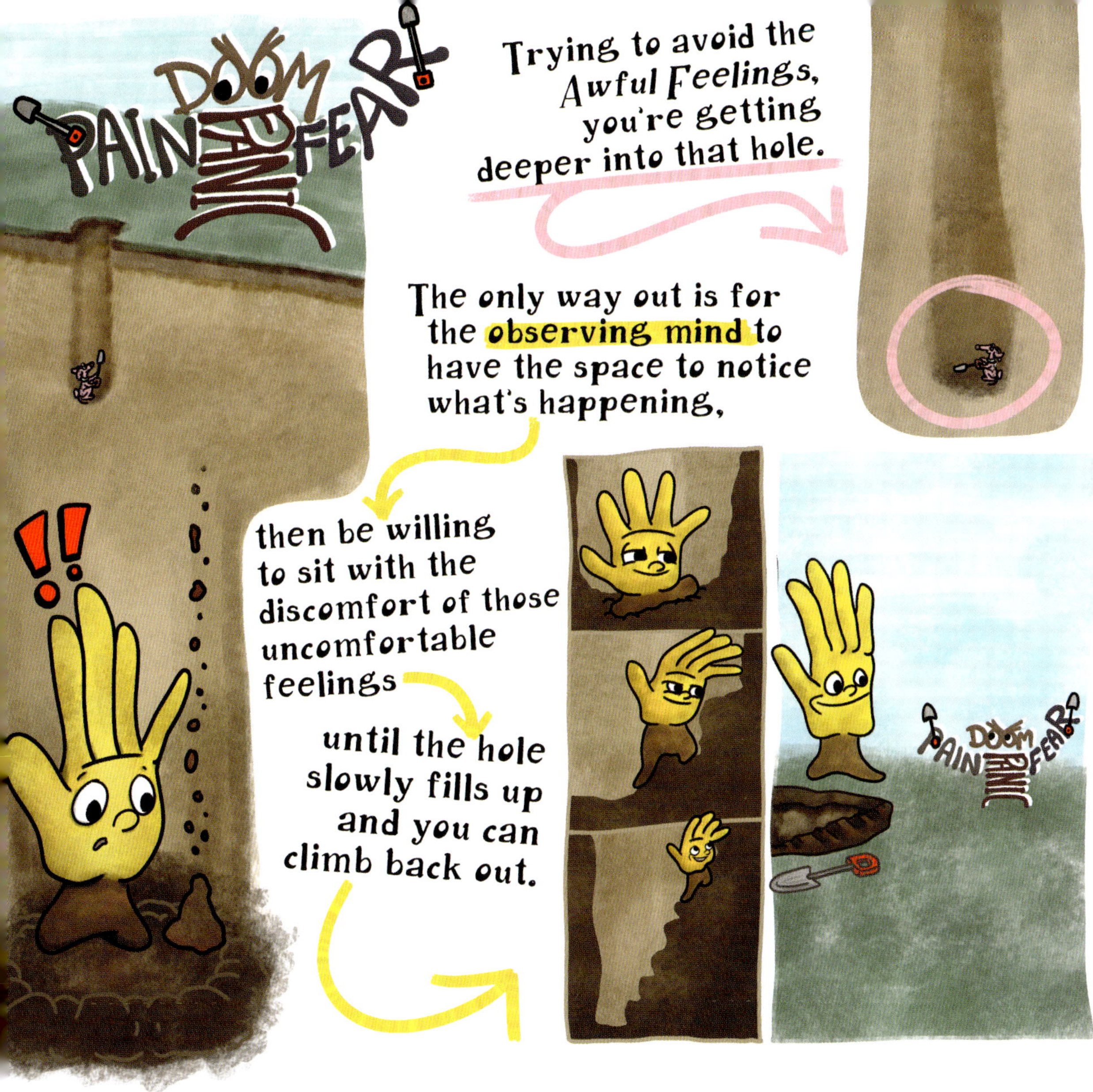
DOOM
PAIN
PANIC
FEAR
Trying to avoid the Awful Feelings, you're getting deeper into that hole.
The only way out is for the observing mind to have the space to notice what's happening,
then be willing to sit with the discomfort of those uncomfortable feelings
until the hole slowly fills up and you can climb back out.
DOOM
PAIN
PANIC
FEAR

It sounds like you want me to deliberately subject myself to pain.

Right now, your best idea has been choosing to avoid the discomfort. That choice is already causing you pain. Pain that's stopping you from enjoying your life and doing things you'd otherwise want to do.

I don't recognise life before all this pain, and I can't imagine having a life like that again. But if I can't stand these feelings, what am I supposed to do other than avoid them?

It can start with "So What?", by accepting those feelings,

and the "Now What?" can then make room for those feelings

so you can start moving towards a goal you value.

For example, the **"So What?"** is to get the **observing self** involved and accept that:

"Hey, this

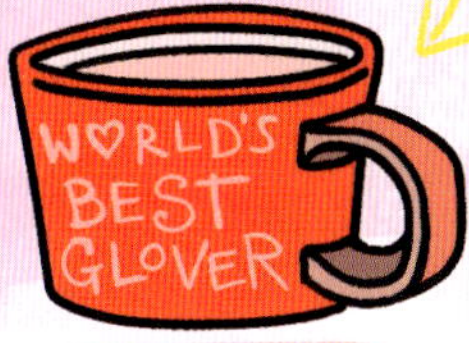

coffee cup from my ex

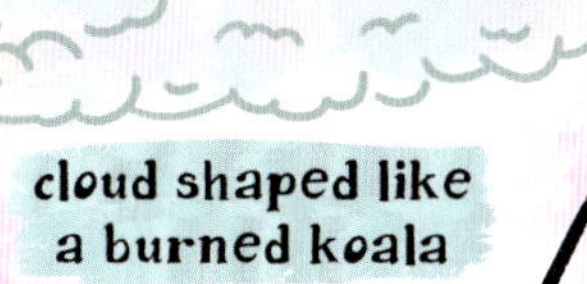

/ cloud shaped like a burned koala /

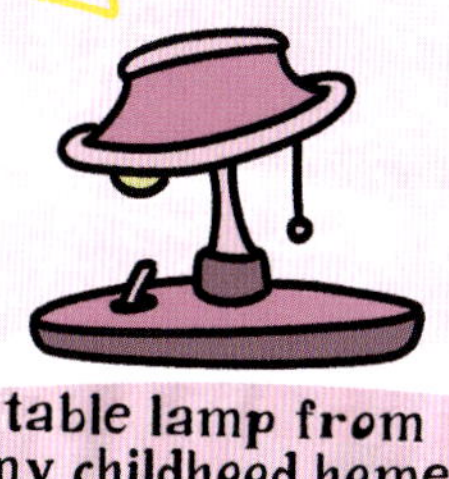

table lamp from my childhood home

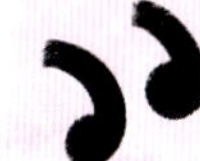

" just set off a **whole cascade** of **painful thoughts** in me.

The **"Now What?"** is to be **curious** about those thoughts and feelings.

Where in your body are they?

Do they move fast or slow?

Do they have a colour, a shape, a temperature?

If you like, take a deep breath and let it out very slowly, like you're blowing up a huge balloon, making space around that feeling.

You'd be surprised how much room we have to feel like this and take a step towards a goal we value.

And that is supposed to *work*?

Only if you're willing to move towards a goal you value with those uncomfortable thoughts and feelings still there.

Sometimes they go away, sometimes they linger.

Yet it's important we keep moving towards our goals, no matter how small the steps are.

And I'm expected to just **carry on** with all this **chaos** happening inside me?

This is where the willingness to move is important.
You can stay stuck in the pain you're in,
or you can make space for this feeling
and take a step towards what you value,
knowing that you will cope.

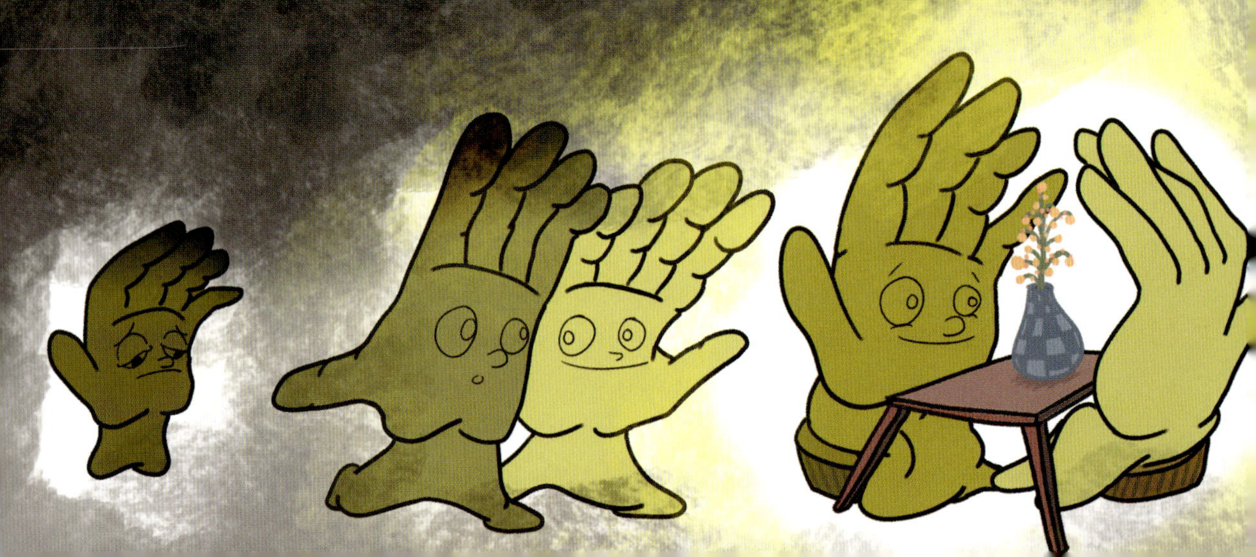

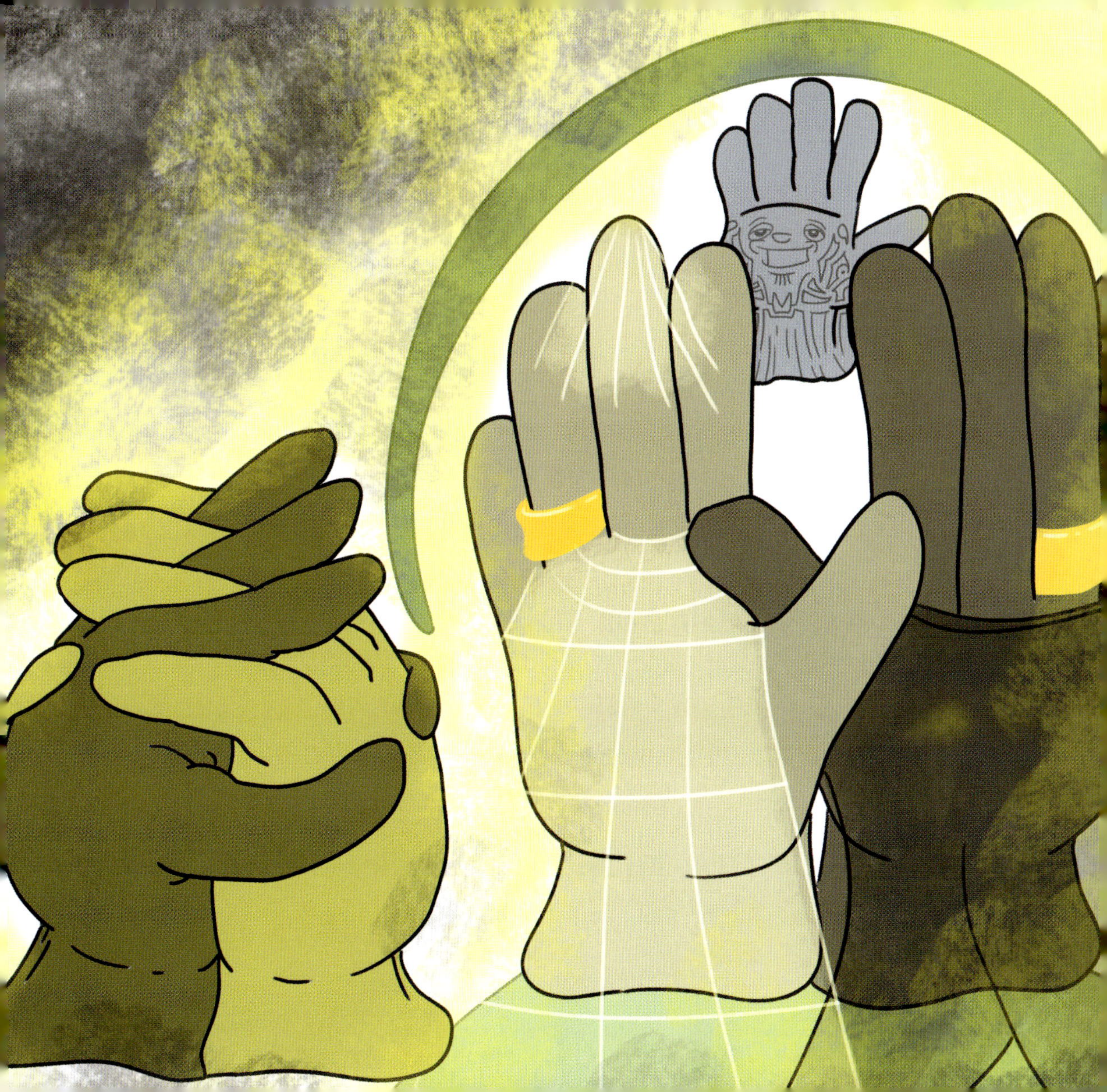

But the thoughts keep coming back.
Over and over and over again.

If we're really stuck, it's important to go and speak to a doctor.

Sometimes we need a little extra help to loosen up the stuck thoughts in our brains so we can make different choices.

What? You want me to take drugs?!!

Don't ask me, I'm a glove not your doctor. Though I do know that medication doesn't **magically make everything better.**

However, it can make it easier to do the work **that makes it better.**

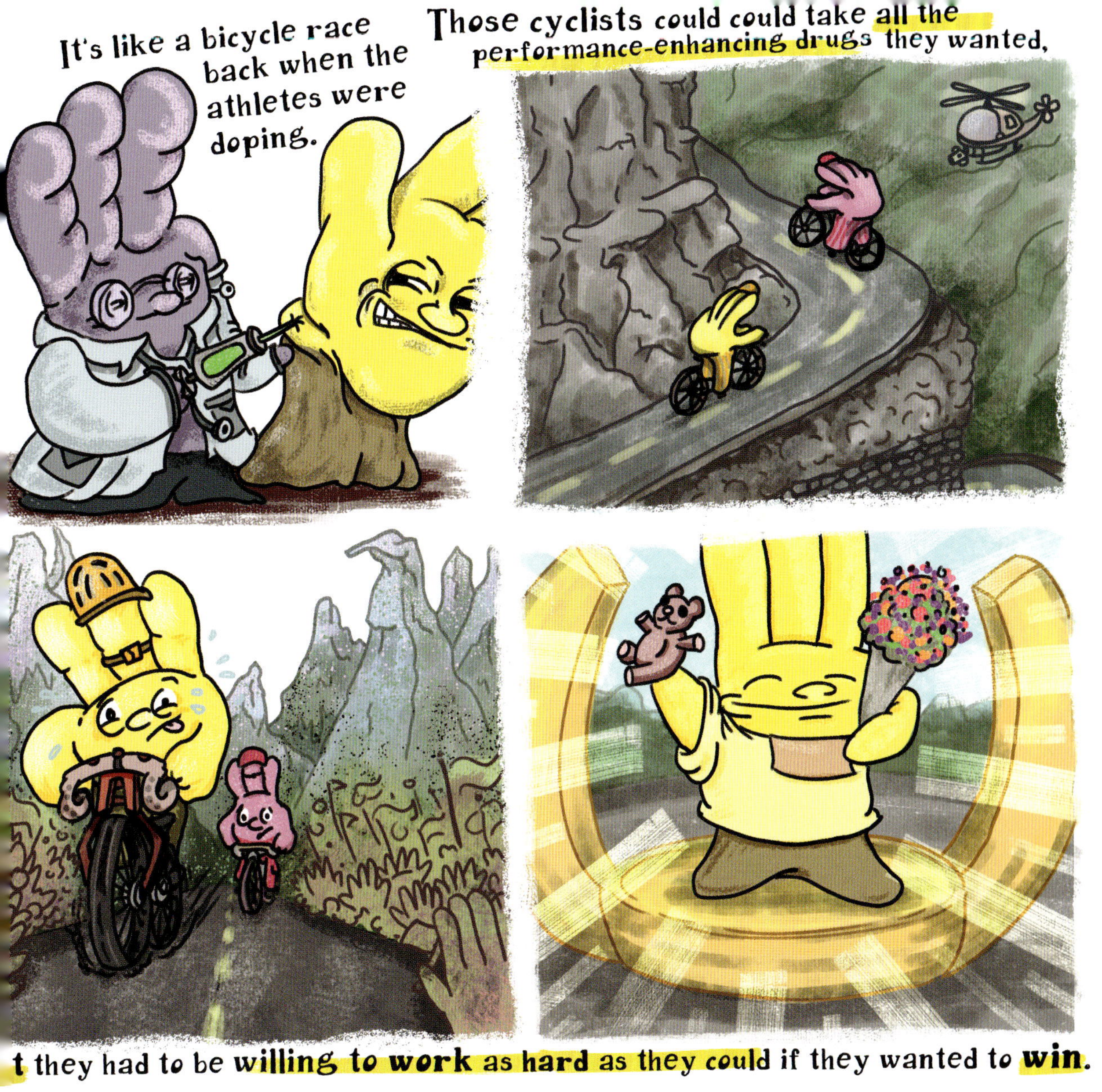

It's like a bicycle race back when the athletes were doping.

Those cyclists could could take all the performance-enhancing drugs they wanted,

t they had to be **willing to work as hard** as they could if they wanted to **win**.

And what does that work look like when it comes to these thoughts?

They won't leave me alone, and the more I push them away the worse they get.

Sometimes it helps to make fun of them. Try giving each particular thought a silly superhero name.

Put them in a ridiculous costume with their underpants on the outside. What's a name you could give to one of your unhelpful thoughts?

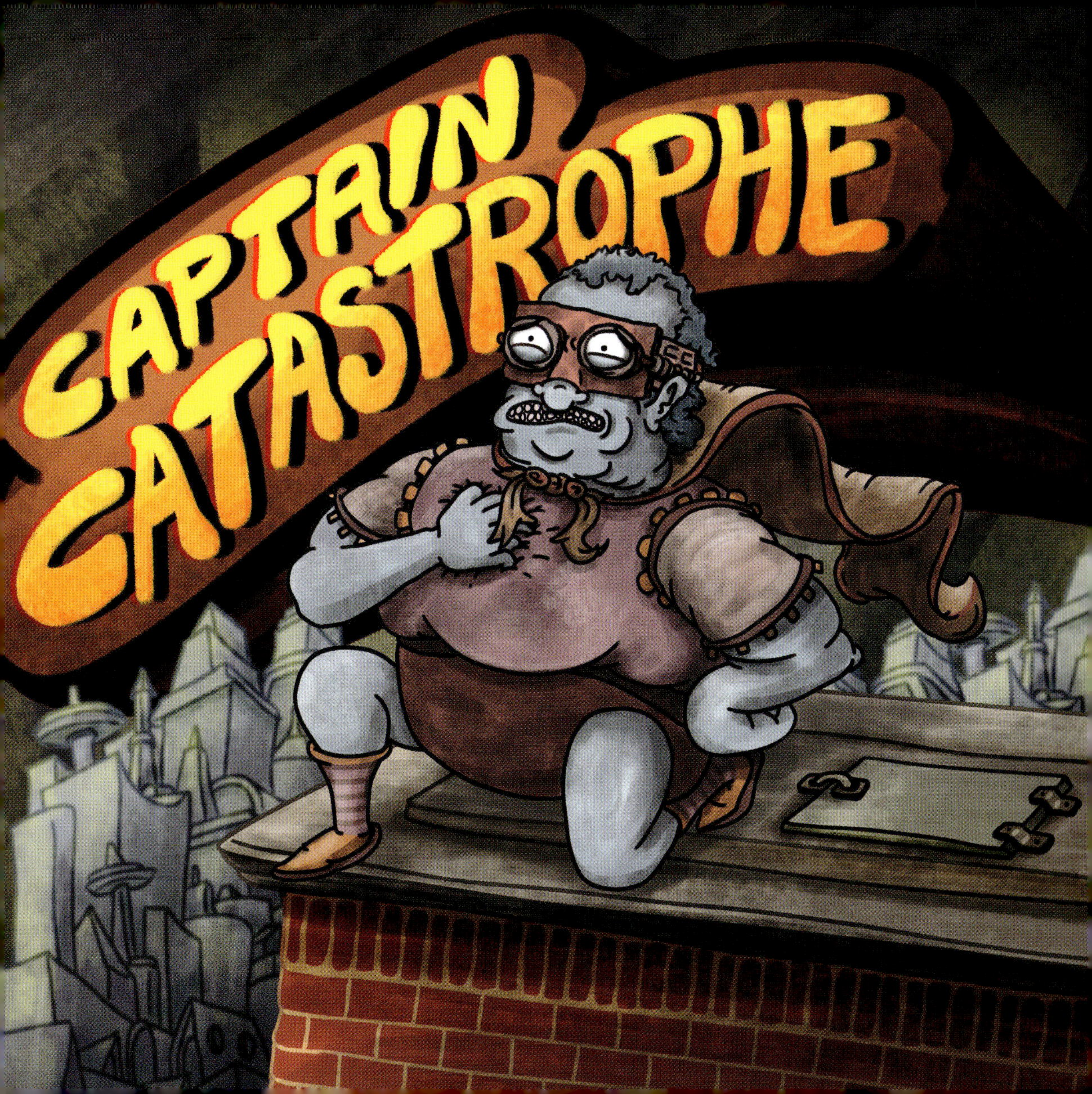
CAPTAIN
CATASTROPHE

There's a **thought** that runs away from me all the time, "**If only**" or "**What if?**".

I guess I could call that thought...
"***Iffy McIffington***"?

A massive, 300kg, kilted cranky rabbit...
that screams in a Scottish accent
"**Och, if only**" or "**Aye, but what if?**"

That's it!

Next time Iffy tries to drag you into an imagined past or frighten you with a made-up future, try to remember that pushing the thoughts away just makes them stronger.

Instead, try saying to yourself

"Thanks, Iffy McIffington. I know you're trying to protect me, but I'm perfectly safe doing what I'm doing."

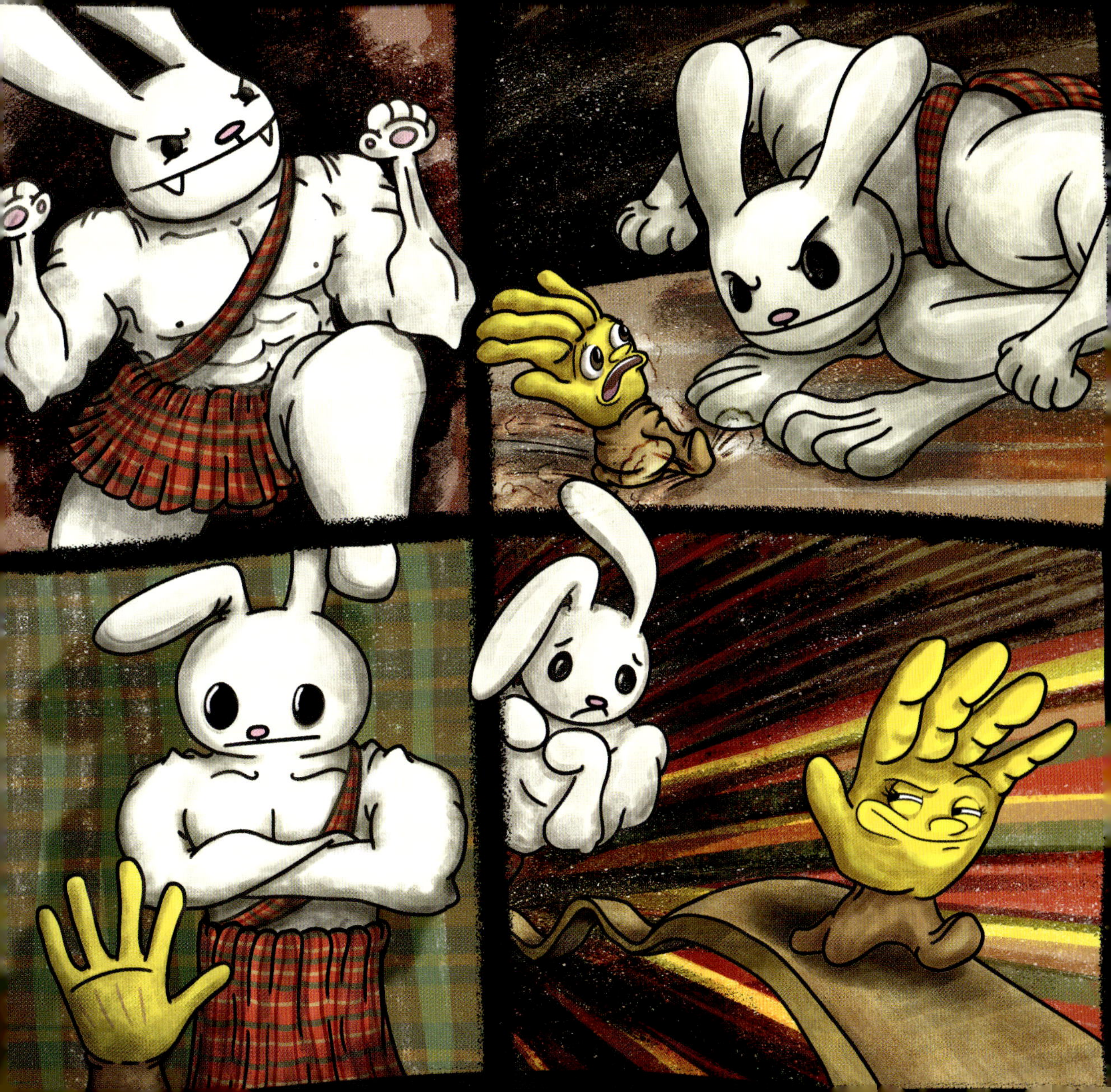

Okay, but where am I going to?

As long as you're moving away from the pain and towards a goal you value, you're doing perfectly.

It doesn't even matter how small the steps are, just be willing to keep moving.

If you value your family but haven't talked to one of them in many years,

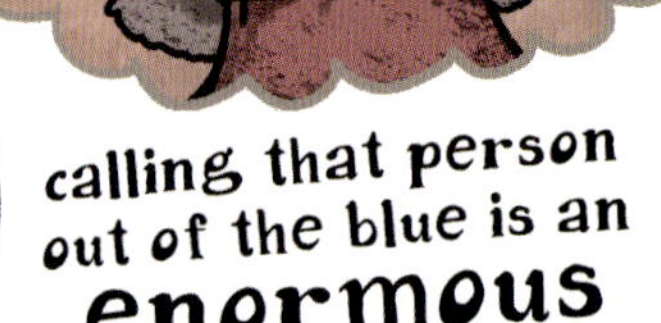

calling that person out of the blue is an **enormous** step to take.

The idea can feel so **overwhelming** that we end up not doing ***anything.***

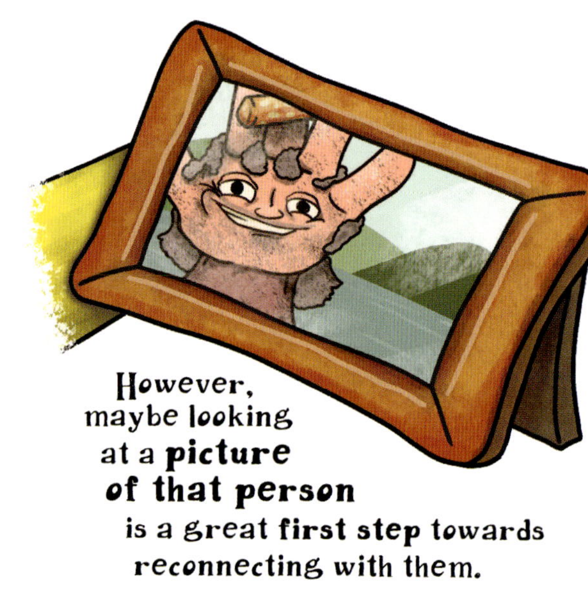

However, maybe looking at a **picture of that person** is a great **first step** towards reconnecting with them.

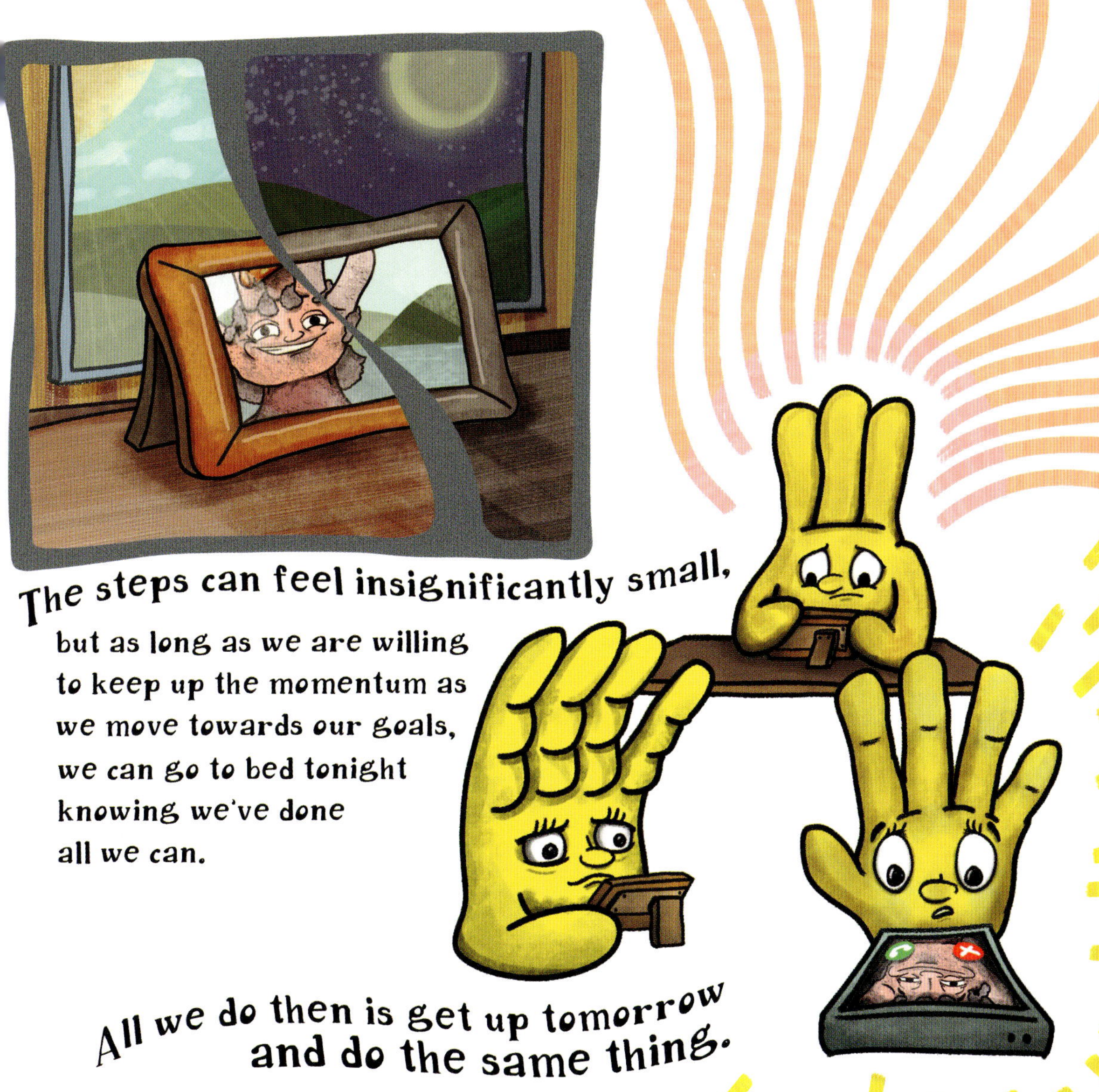

The steps can feel insignificantly small,

but as long as we are willing to keep up the momentum as we move towards our goals, we can go to bed tonight knowing we've done all we can.

All we do then is get up tomorrow and do the same thing.

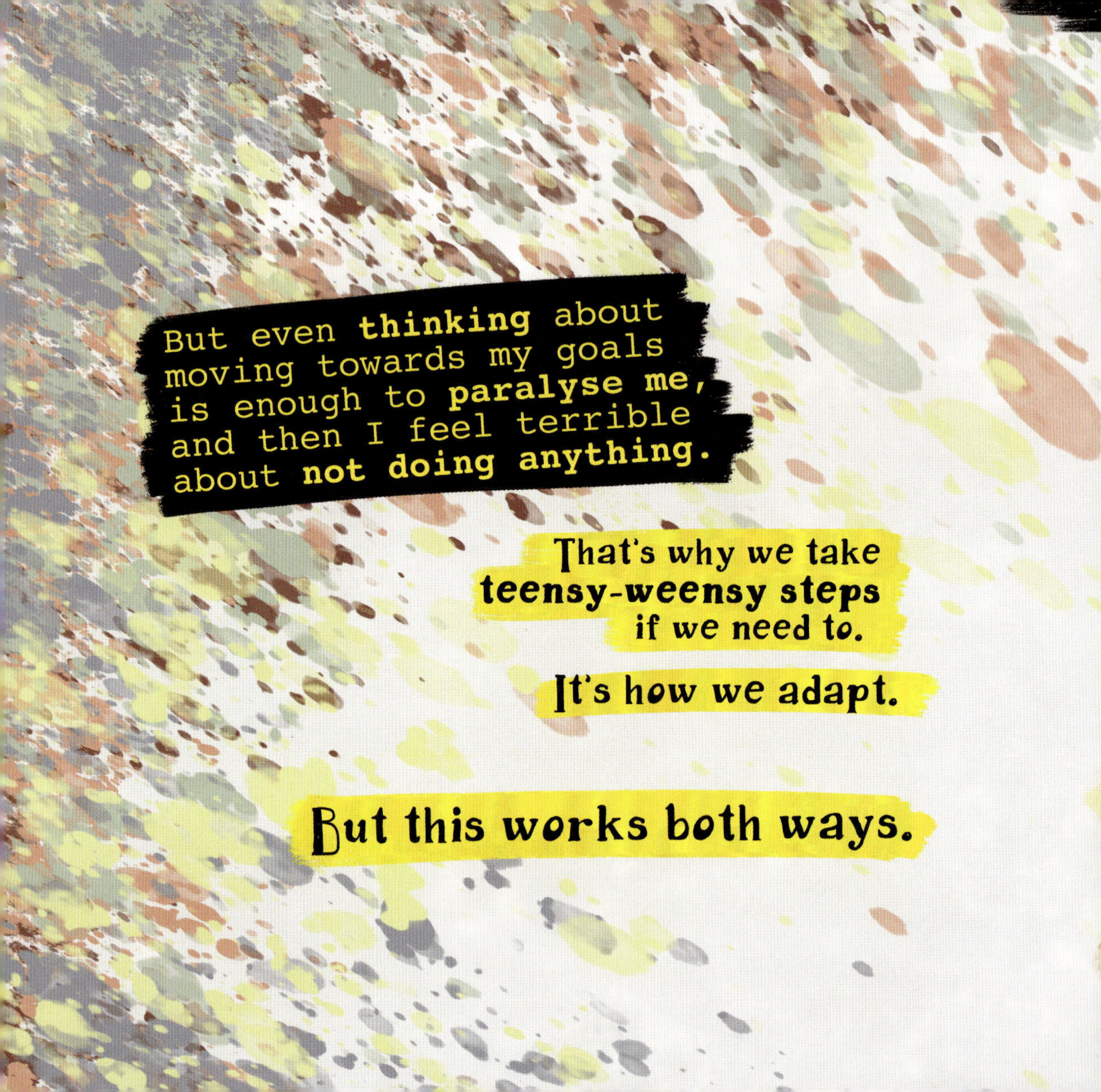
But even **thinking** about moving towards my goals is enough to **paralyse me**, and then I feel terrible about **not doing anything**.
That's why we take **teensy-weensy steps** if we need to.
It's how we adapt.
But this works both ways.

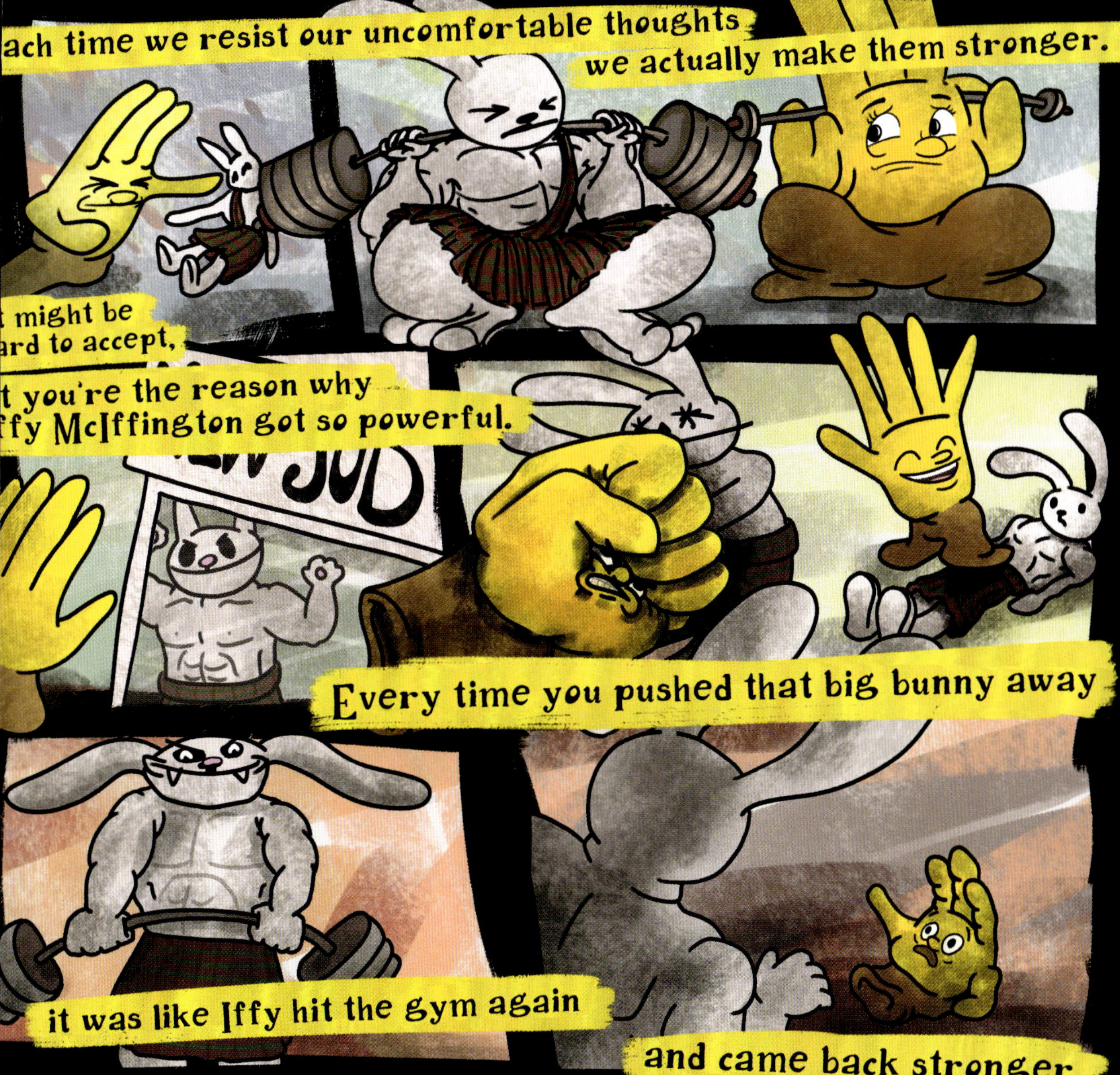

ach time we resist our uncomfortable thoughts
we actually make them stronger.
t might be
ard to accept,
t you're the reason why
ffy McIffington got so powerful.
Every time you pushed that big bunny away
it was like Iffy hit the gym again
and came back stronger.

So by training my **ability** to be with the **discomfort**,
I'm making myself stronger too?

Exactly.
The discomfort might go away,

then again
it might not.

We don't want the discomfort to go away altogether, because uncomfortable thoughts and feelings are an important part of what makes us human.

We learn from them, and more importantly, we grow from them. If we can build up our ability to handle them, we make room for the life we want to live.

A life that involves joy, achievement, love, happiness and fulfilment.

This sounds like a *lot of work*,
and I'm **so burned out** from living like this.
I don't know if I'm strong enough.

You're already strong enough to handle what has been unbelievably hard for you.

You're so determined and persistent, because you keep choosing similar responses to your discomfort even though you're not getting the results you want.

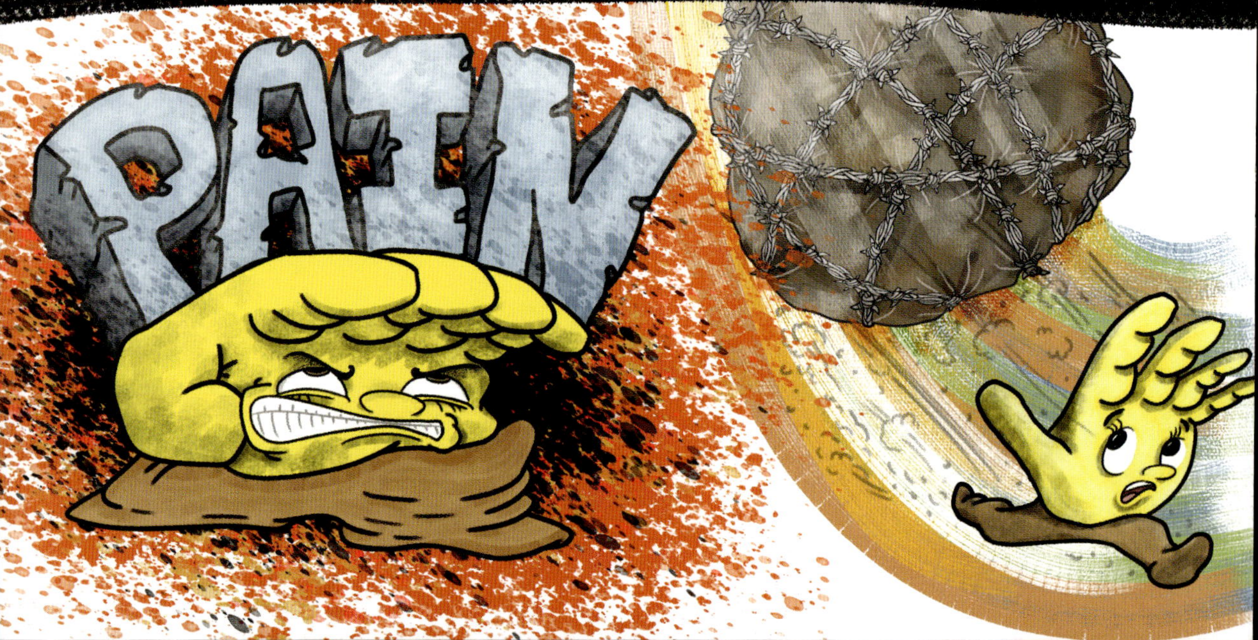

You have already proven to yourself that you have the strength, determination and persistence needed to consistently make tough choices.

Which is lucky, because choosing acceptance and action can be tough.

But every time you make that choice you win. We build a rich life full of purpose and meaning one choice at a time.

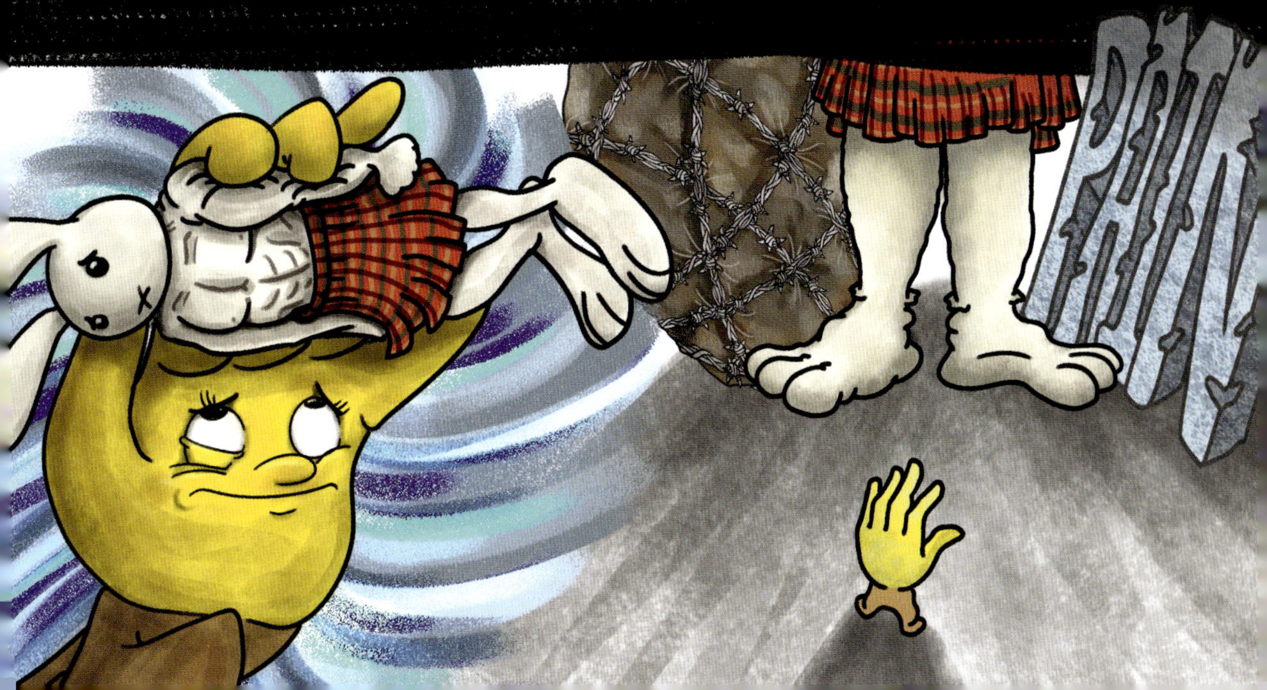

But what about the things I'm frightened about **in the future?**

War, suffering, climate chaos, **massive global stuff that I can't control.**

Those things can be really frightening.

It's important to remind yourself that even
with all of the pain you've been dealing with,
you're only here today
because in some way
you have managed to cope with
every challenge you've ever faced.
Why would it be any different in the future?

You're very optimistic, aren't you?

Not really. I'm just making a *choice* about how I look at it.

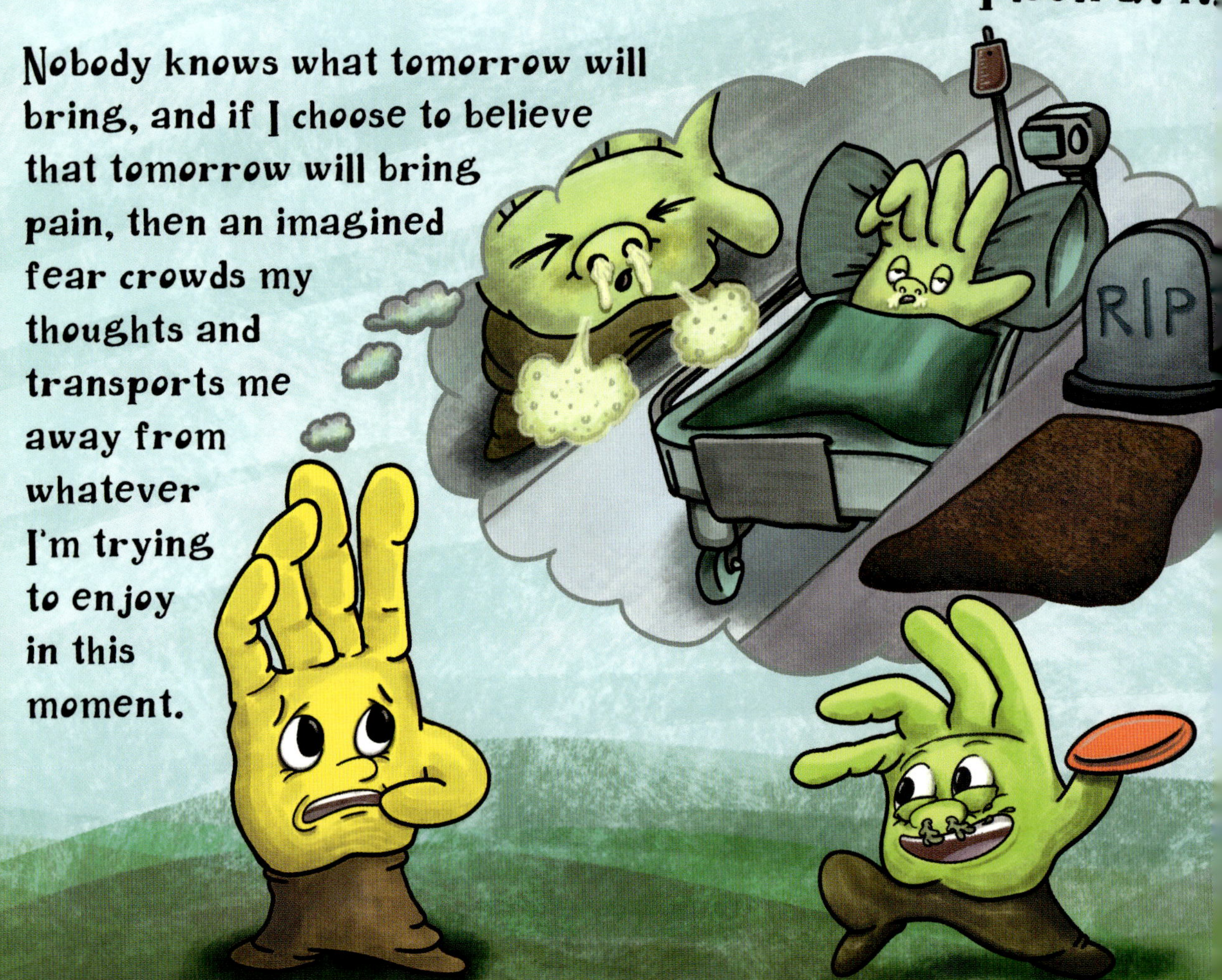

Nobody knows what tomorrow will bring, and if I choose to believe that tomorrow will bring pain, then an imagined fear crowds my thoughts and transports me away from whatever I'm trying to enjoy in this moment.

It's all a choice.

I can choose to react to what my mind is predicting,

or I can choose to react to what's happening in this moment, trusting that I can handle it.

I know this is true because so far I've been able to cope with every single challenging thing those moments have brought.

This frees me up to be here in the moment with you, and the moment is all we ever have.

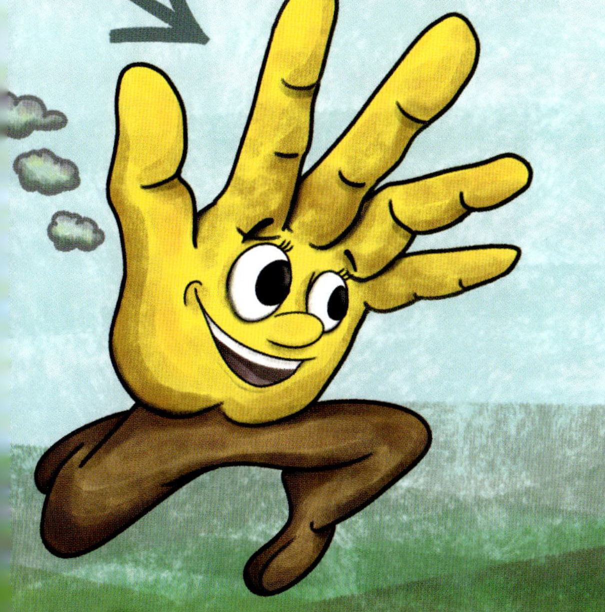

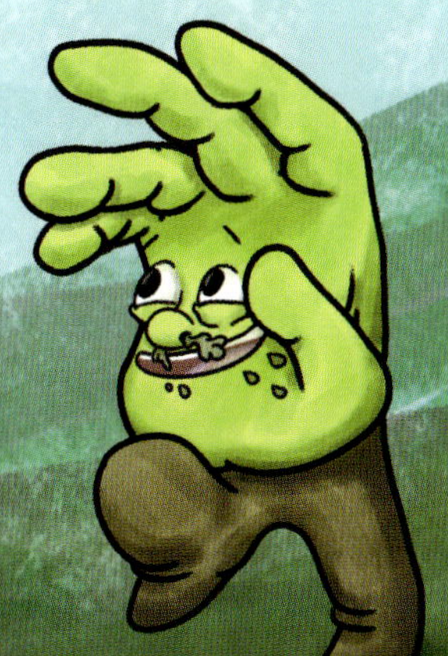

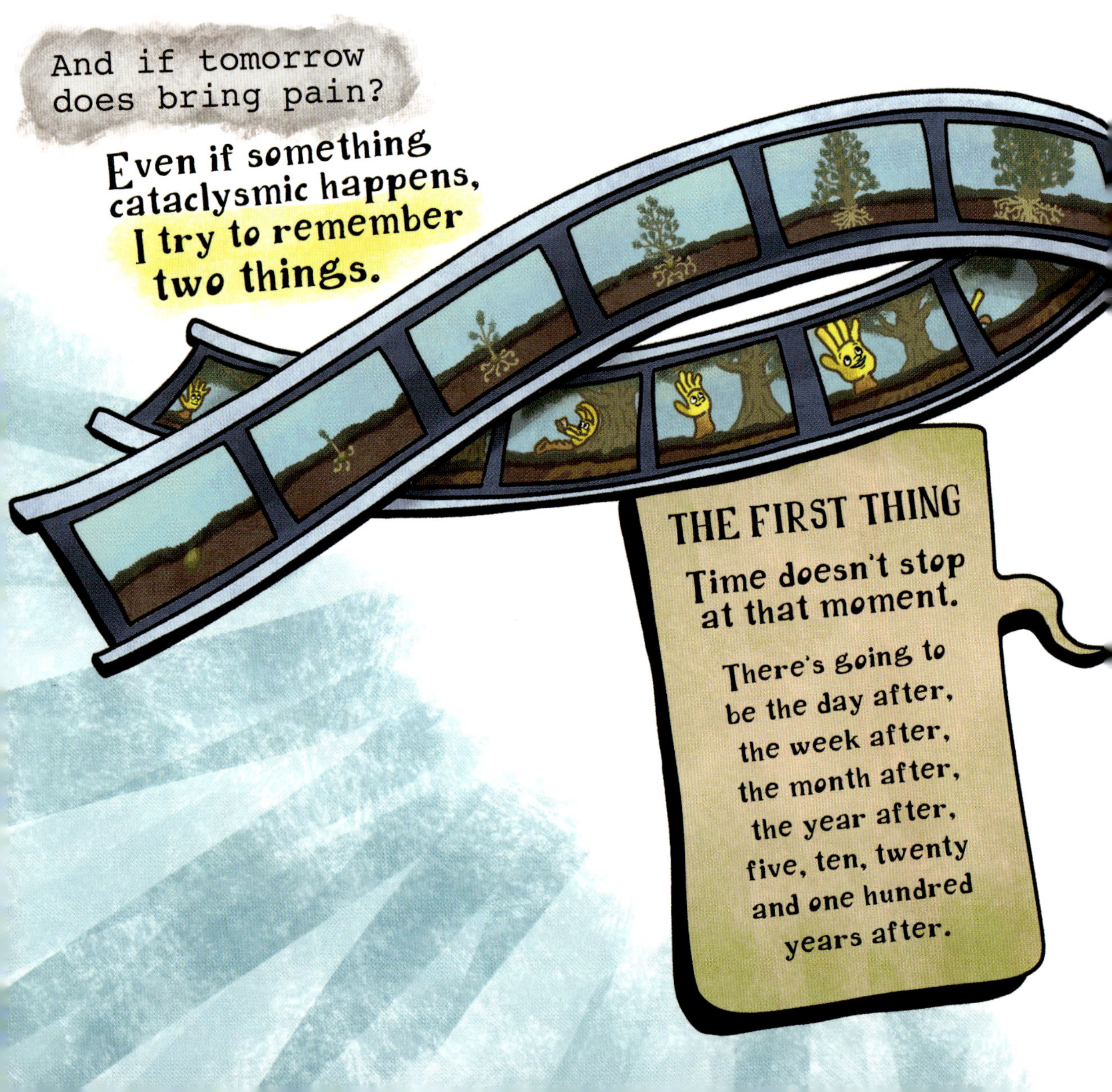
And if tomorrow does bring pain?
Even if something cataclysmic happens, I try to remember two things.
THE FIRST THING
Time doesn't stop at that moment.
There's going to be the day after, the week after, the month after, the year after, five, ten, twenty and one hundred years after.

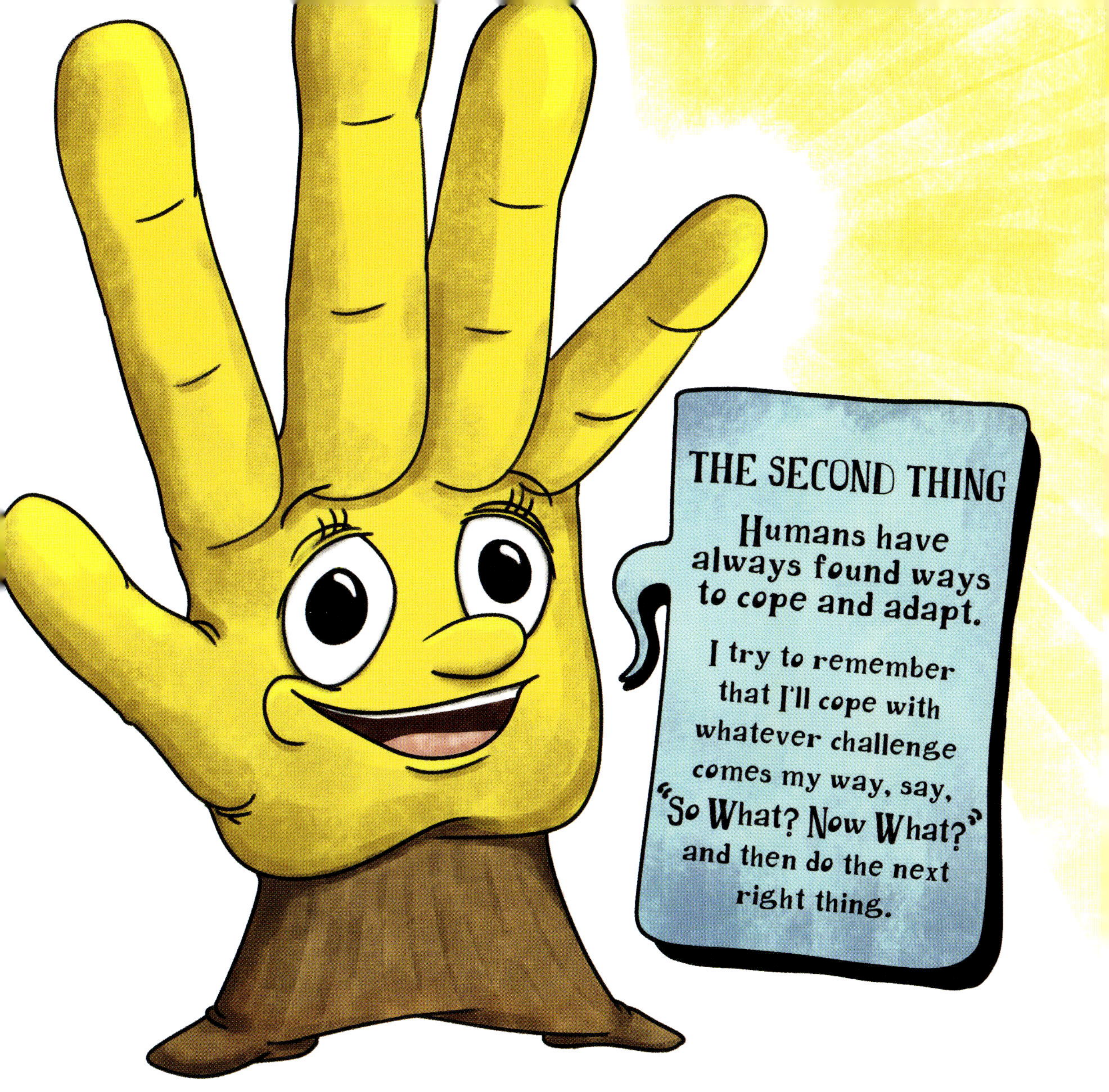
THE SECOND THING
Humans have always found ways to cope and adapt.
I try to remember that I'll cope with whatever challenge comes my way, say, "So What? Now What?" and then do the next right thing.

And what's the next right thing for me?

The willingness to take the **smallest step** towards a goal that you value.

Then being willing to take another.

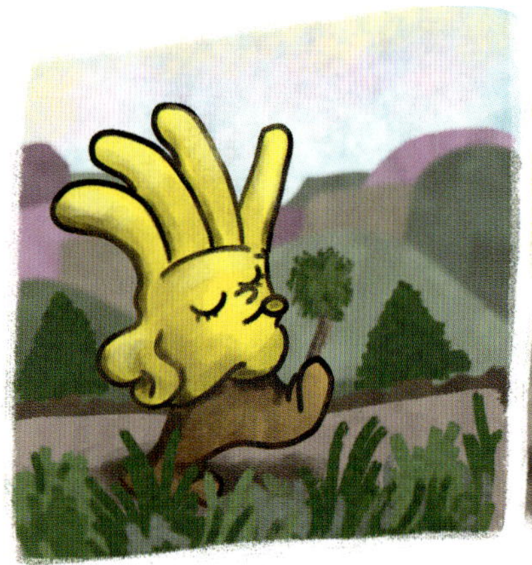

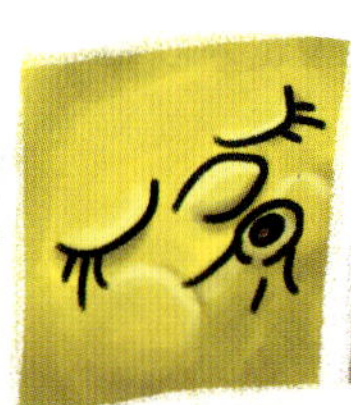

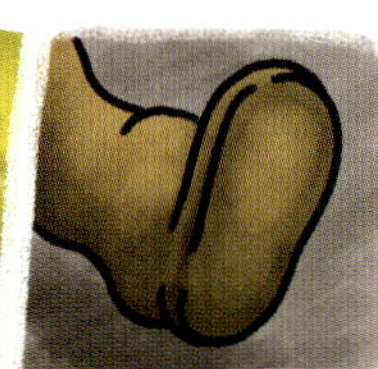

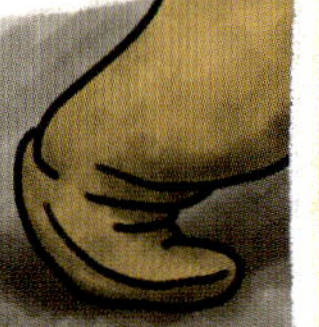

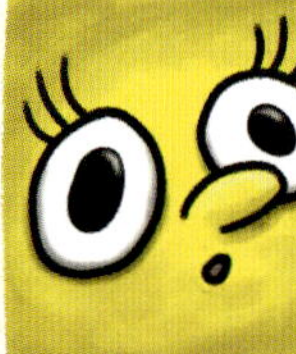

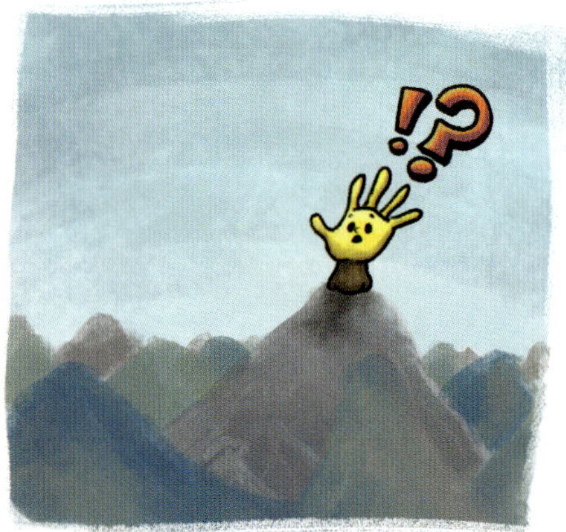

You don't just wander around and accidentally end up at the top of a mountain.

It takes deliberate action, step by step by step.

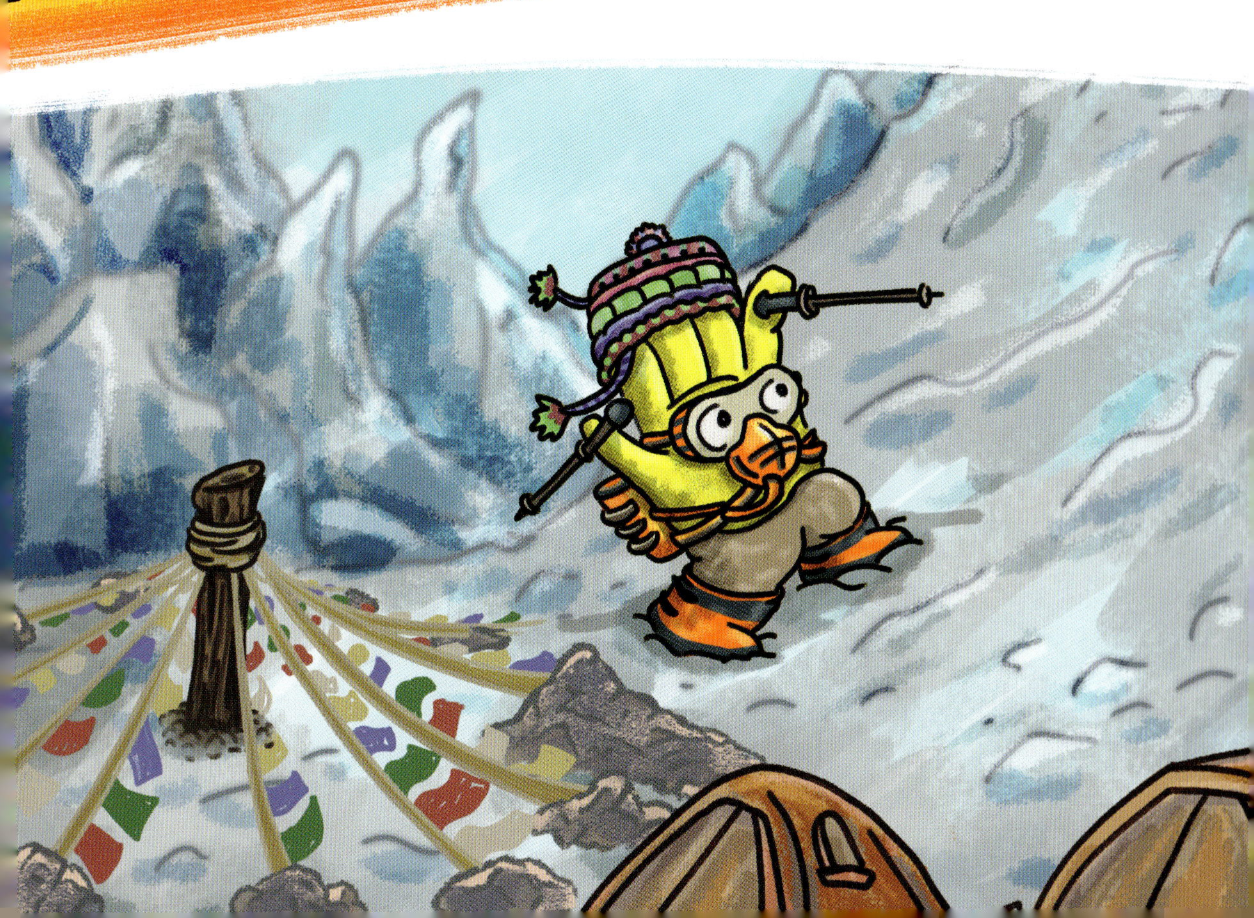

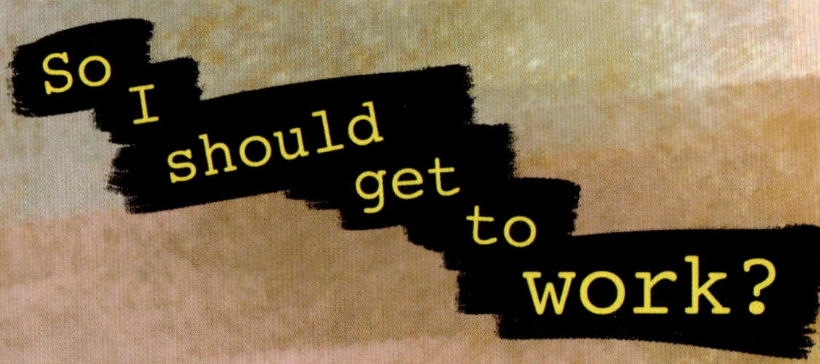
So I should get to work?

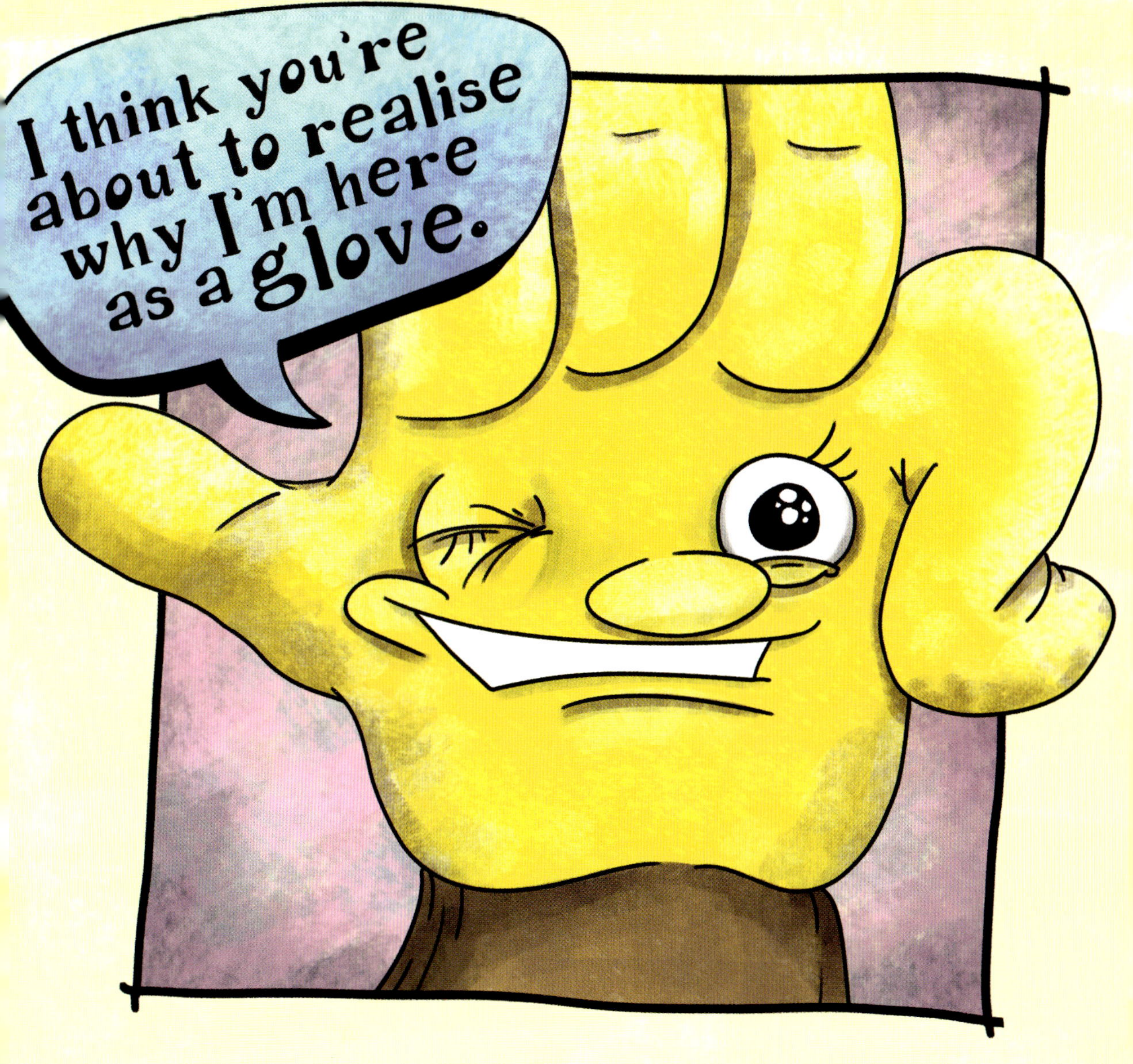
I think you're about to realise why I'm here as a glove.

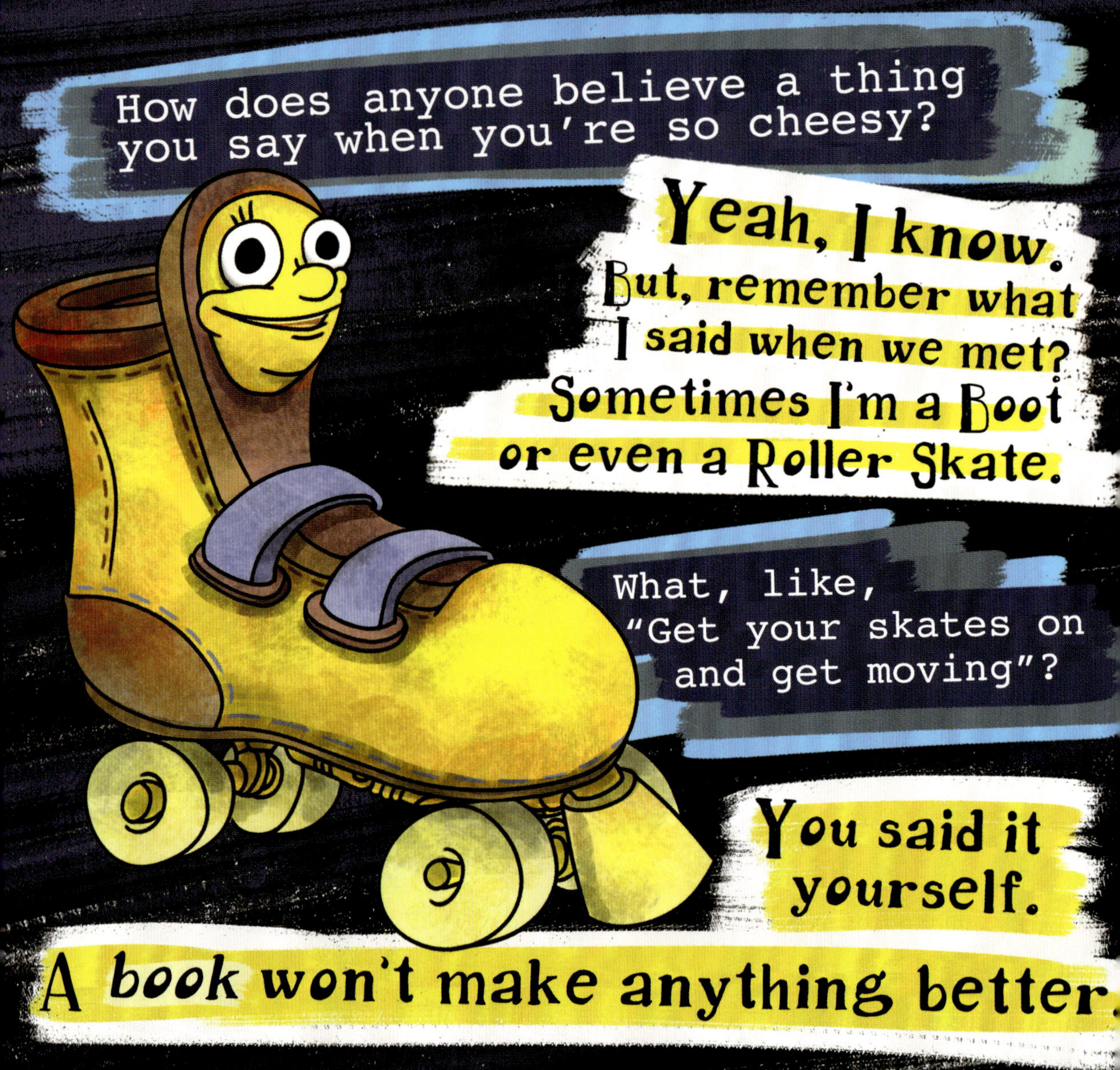
How does anyone believe a thing you say when you're so cheesy?
Yeah, I know. But, remember what I said when we met? Sometimes I'm a Boot or even a Roller Skate.
What, like, "Get your skates on and get moving"?
You said it yourself.
A *book* won't make anything better.

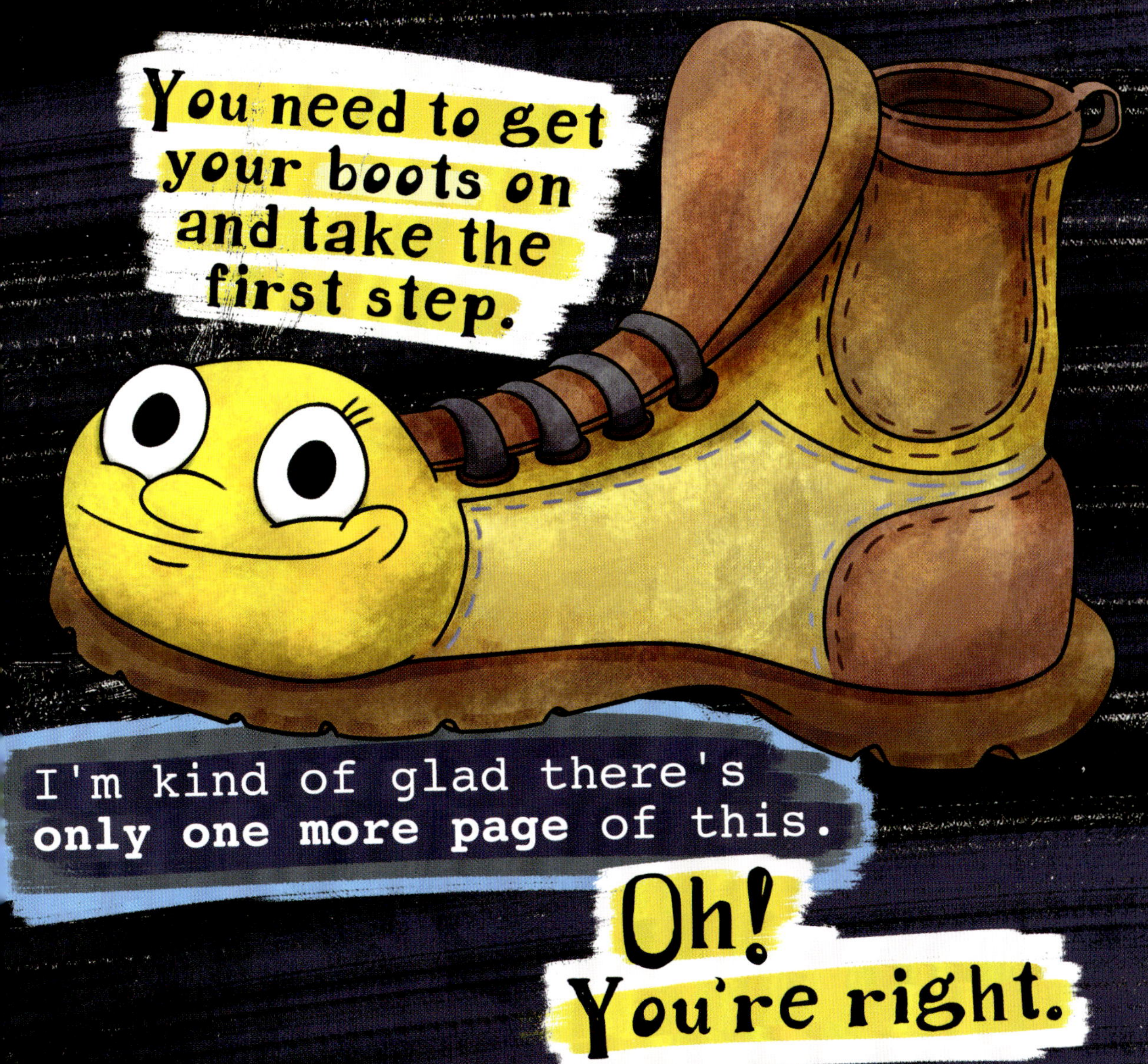
You need to get your boots on and take the first step.
I'm kind of glad there's only one more page of this.
Oh! You're right.

I guess you'd better pull your gloves on and ...

...get to work?

Exactly!

Oh, that's so lame.

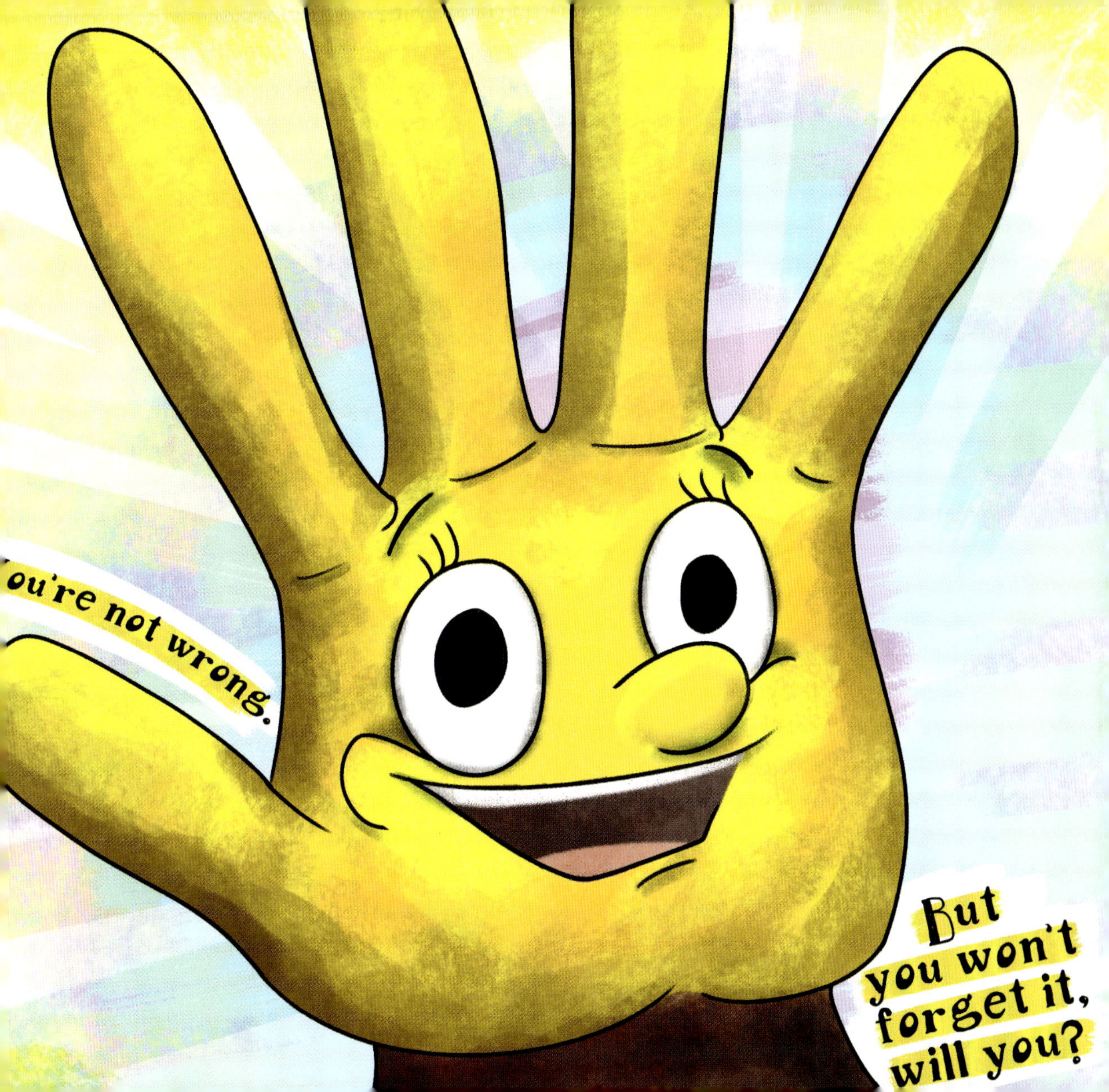
ou're not wrong.
But
you won't
forget it,
will you?

Acknowledgements

OG would like to thank Brandon VanOver at Penguin Random House for believing in this book, Ben Richardson for the business guidance, David S for the spiritual guidance and all of his shrinks for the mental guidance.

He'd like to thank the eminent psychologist Julie Grove, who, along with making sure every page in this book is accurate, had to figure out if a dog in a hole was an accurate representation of an otherwise complex psychological concept. (Turns out it is.)

He'd like to thank Campbell Walker for being such an inspiring human being and a dream collaborator.

He'd also like to thank his DNA family, his Sobriety family, his work family and mostly his actual family, Audrey, Georgia and Wolfie, for making the "Now What?" a simple question to answer.

Cam would like to thank Milo, Zelda, and Felicity. A lot.
Same to his Mum and the rest of his whānau.

He'd like to thank Osher for his warmth, wisdom and wicked-sick earth-shatteringly infectious mega-growth-provoking mindset.

Finally, he'd like to thank the team at Penguin as well as the real penguins he saw at the aquarium with his kids on the weekend. One group of penguins represents family, and the other penguins creativity: the two answers to "Now What?" that truly make his life worth living.

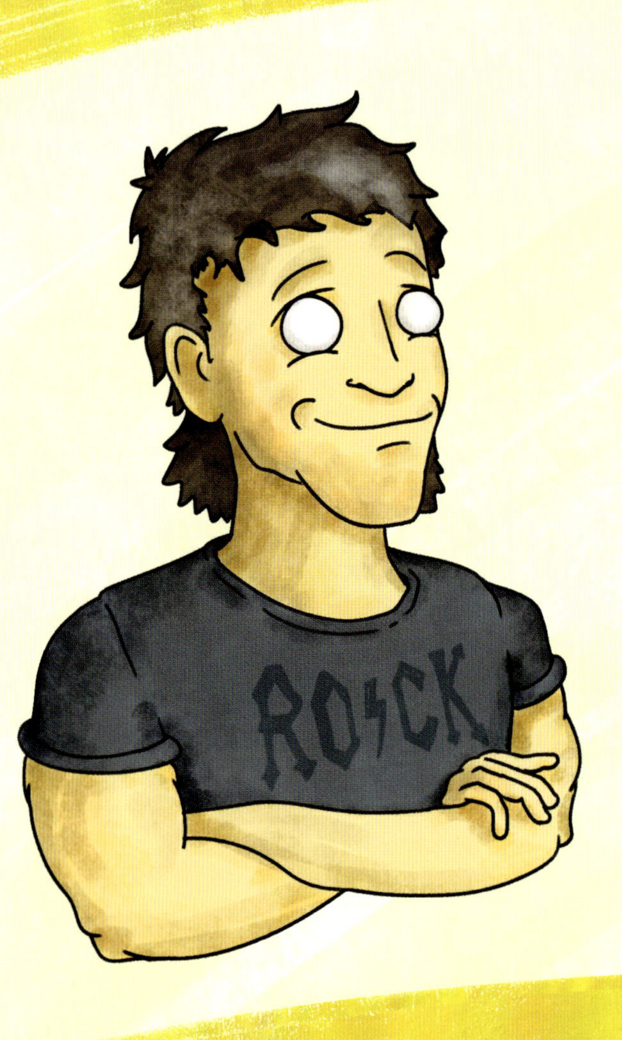
ROCK

OSHER GÜNSBERG is a multifaceted Australian media figure, renowned as a television host (*Australian Idol*, *The Bachelor* franchise, *The Masked Singer*), the host of the acclaimed podcast *Better Than Yesterday*, which has been running weekly since 2013, and an in-demand keynote speaker. His career began in Brisbane radio before moving to music television in the 2000s, making him a familiar presence across generations.

He is also the bestselling author of the ABIA-nominated memoir *Back, After the Break* (HarperCollins, 2018) and an award-winning documentary maker, celebrated for *A Matter of Life and Death* and *A World of Pain*. Passionate about positive change, Osher is a vocal advocate for mental health and climate action.

He currently lives in Sydney with his family, but will always go for Queensland in the State of Origin.

CAMPBELL WALKER is the bestselling author of *Your Head is a Houseboat* and *Doom and Bloom*, as well as an illustrator, animator and content creator, better known as Struthless. His YouTube channel has amassed over 1 million subscribers and 50 million views across topics such as mental health, sociology and creativity.

Cam has worked with Comedy Central, Spotify, Vice, Shopify, GQ, The Betoota Advocate, Tinder, Samsung, Gatorade and Universal Music. Before he pursued his passion - writing and illustrating - Cam worked as an advertising creative director, a tattooist and (for one very strange week) a golf-cart taxi driver at a country music festival in Arizona.

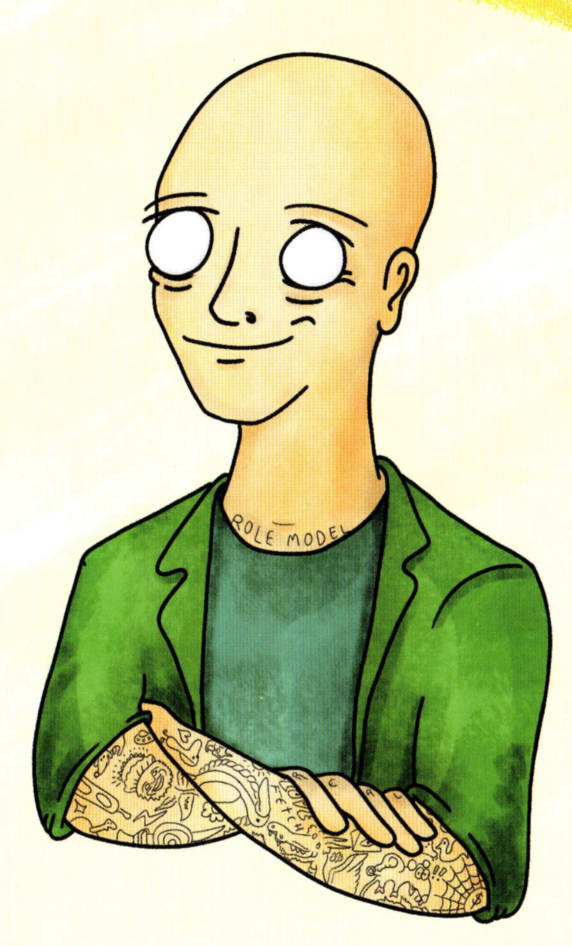
ROLE MODEL

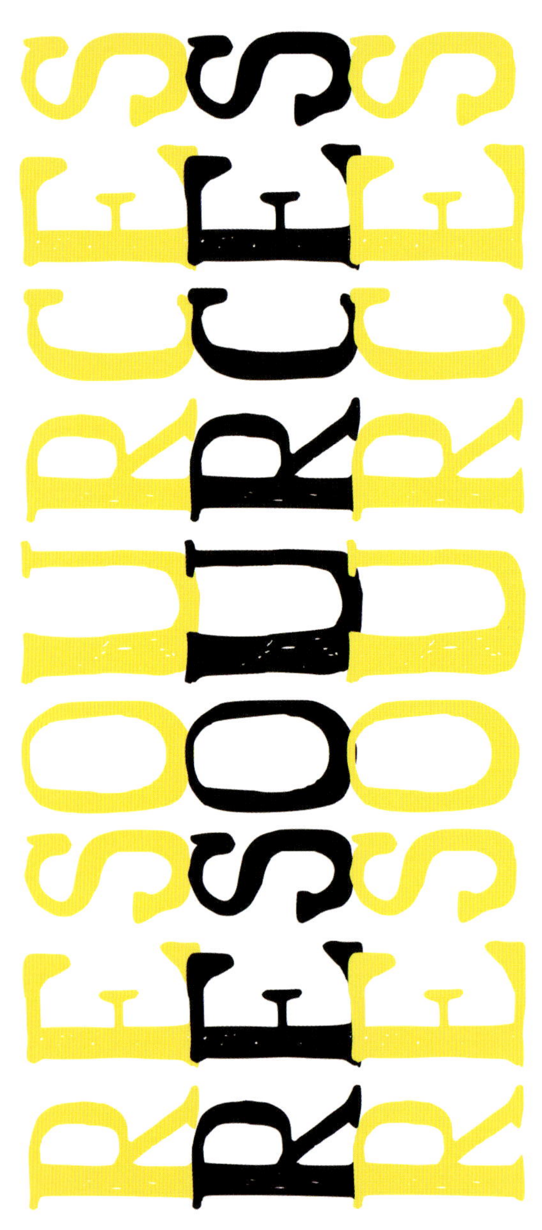

24-hour crisis support helplines

Lifeline - 13 11 1 4
lifeline.org.au

Suicide Call Back Service - 1300 659 467
suicidecallbackservice.org.au

Mental health support

Beyond Blue - 1300 224 636
beyondblue.org.au

SANE - 1800 187 263
sane.org

Mensline Australia - 1300 78 99 78
mensline.org.au

Kids Helpline - 1800 55 1800
kidshelpline.com.au

Headspace - 1800 650 890
headspace.org.au

Veterans and families counselling

Open Arms - 1800 011 046
openarms.gov.au

Domestic, family and sexual violence support

1800RESPECT (1800 73 7 732)
1800respect.org.au

Drug and alcohol support

National Alcohol and Other Drug Hotline
1800 250 015
health.gov.au/our-work/drug-help

Gambling support

Gamblers Help - 1800 858 858
gamblershelp.com.au

Complex trauma support

BlueKnot - 1300 657 380
blueknot.org.au

Eating disorders and body image support

Butterfly Foundation
1800 33 4673
butterfly.org.au

Post/perinatal support

PANDA- 1300 726 306
panda.org.au

LGBTQ+ support

QLife - 1800 184 527
qlife.org.au

Crisis support for Aboriginal and Torres Strait Islander people

13Yarn - 13 92 76
13yarn.org.au

SO WHAT?

PENGUIN BOOKS

UK | USA | Canada | Ireland | Australia
India | New Zealand | South Africa | China

Penguin Books is part of the Penguin Random House group of companies whose addresses can be found at global.penguinrandomhouse.com

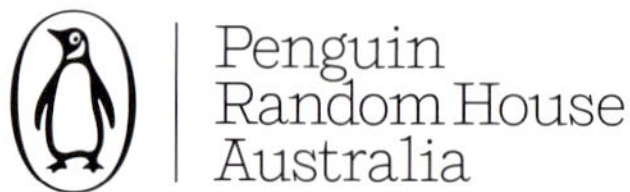

First published by Penguin Books in 2025

Internal illustration, design and typesetting by Campbell Walker
Cover design by Campbell Walker © Penguin Random House Australia Pty Ltd

Printed and bound in China by 1010 Printing International Co Ltd.

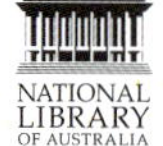

A catalogue record for this book is available from the National Library of Australia

ISBN 978 1 76135 230 0

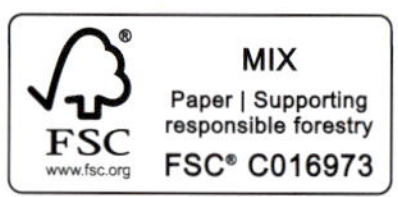

We at Penguin Random House Australia acknowledge that Aboriginal and Torres Strait Islander peoples are the Traditional Custodians and the first storytellers of the lands on which we live and work. We honour Aboriginal and Torres Strait Islander peoples' continuous connection to Country, waters, skies and communities. We celebrate Aboriginal and Torres Strait Islander stories, traditions and living cultures, and we pay our respects to Elders past and present.